Thai Massage
Workbook

Second Edition,
Fully Revised and Updated

Companion Book Available

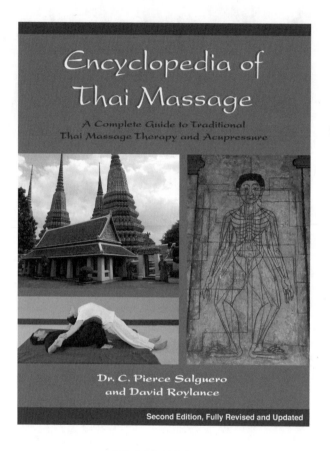

978-1-84409-563-3

available from your local bookstore,
or directly from publisher at

www.findhornpress.com

Thai Massage Workbook

David Roylance

and

Dr. C. Pierce Salguero

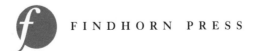
FINDHORN PRESS

First published by Findhorn Press 2007. Second edition, fully revised and updated, published by Findhorn Press 2011.

ISBN: 978-1-84409-564-3

British Library Cataloguing-in-Publication Data.
A catalogue record for this book is available from the British Library.

Massage photography by Keith Edwards of Statesider Photography
(www.statesider.com), ©2011 David Roylance.
Special thanks to our models Viengkhong Khambay and Ketsarin Phaopanfeung,
who volunteered their hard work for this book.
Anatomical drawings ©2001-2011 David O. Schuster

Cover design by Richard Crookes
Interior design by Damian Keenan
Printed and bound in the USA

1 2 3 4 5 6 7 8 9 10 20 19 18 17 16 15 14 13 12 11

Published by
Findhorn Press
117-121 High Street,
Forres IV36 1AB Scotland,
United Kingdom

t +44-(0)1309-690582
f +44(0)131-777-2711
e info@findhornpress.com
www.findhornpress.com

Contents

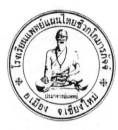

Shivagakomarpaj Lineage "Wai Khru"
(Ceremony Honoring the Teacher)
Dedicated to Jivaka Komarabhacca,
Founder of Thai Medicine

ไหว้ครู

บทนมัสการพระชีวกโกมารภัจจ
(ผู้ค้นพบการแพทย์แผนไทย)
โอม นะโม ชีวะโก สิระสา
อะหัง กรุณิโก สัพพะสัตตานัง
โอสะถะ ทิพพะมันตัง ปะภาโส
สุริยาจันทัง โกมารภัตโต
ปะกาเสสิ วันทามิ ปัณฑิโต
สุเมธะโส อะโรคา สุมะนาโหมิ
(3จบ)

ปิโยเทวะ มะนุสสานัง ปิโยพรหมมา
นะมุตตะโม ปิโยนาคะ สุปันนานัง ปิณินทริยัง
นะมามิหัง นะโมพุทธายะ นะวนนะเวียน
นะสะถิต นะเสถียน เอหิมามา นะเวียนนะแวะ
นะไปทางเวียน นะเวียนมาหากู เอหิมามา
ปิยังมะมะ นะโมพุทธายะ
(1 จบ)

นะมะพะทะ นะโมพทุ ธายะ (3 จบเฉพาะตอนเช้า)

นะอะ นะวะ โรคา พยาธิ วินัสสันติ **(3 จบ)**

มหาลาภา ปิยงัมะมะ (3 จบเฉพาะตอนเช้า)

สาธุ โน ภันเต **(กราบ)**

อาจารย์ เจ้าหน้าที่ ผู้ฝึกงาน และนักเรียน ถวายสังฆทาน

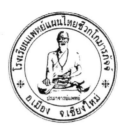

Shivagakomarpaj Lineage "Wai Khru"
(Ceremony Honoring the Teacher)
Dedicated to Jivaka Komarabhacca,
Founder of Thai Medicine

Pronunciation Guide

Ohm-Nā-Mo / Chi-Va-Ko / Si-Ra-Sāā /
Ar-Hāng / Ka-Rū-Nī-Ko / Shap-Phā-Sat-Ta-Nang
Oh-Sa-Tā / Tīp-Pha-Man-Tang / Pa-Pha-Sō /
Su-Ri-Ya-Jan-Thung / Ko-Ma-Ra-Phāt-Toe
Pa-Ka-Say-Si / Won-Ta-Mi / Phan-Ti-Toe /
Su-May-Thā-So / Ah-Ro-Kaa / Su-Ma-Na-Ho-Mī /
(Repeat 3 times)

Pi-Yo-Te-Wā / Ma-Nus-Sa-Nang / Pi-Yo-Phrom-Mā / Na-Mut-Ta-Mo /
Pi-Yo-Na-Ka / Su-Pun-Na-Nang / Pi-Nin-See-Young / Na-Ma-Mi-Hūng /
(Repeat 1 time)

Nā-Mo-Put-Tā-Ya / Nā-Von-Nā-Vean /
Na-Sa-Tit / Na-Sa-Tean / Ey-Hi-Mā-Mā / Na-Vean-Na-Ve /
Na-Pai-Tang-Vean / Na-Vean-Ma-Ha-Kuu / Ey-Hi-Ma-Ma /
Pi-Young-Ma-Ma / Nā-Mo-Put-Tā-Ya
(Repeat 1 time)

Na-Ma-Pa-Ta / Na-Mo-Put-Ta-Yā
(Morning only. Repeat 3 times.)

Na-Ah / Na-Wa / Ro-Kaa / Pa-Yā-Ti / Wi-Nas-Santi
(Repeat 3 times)

Ma-Hā-La-Pa / Pi-Young-Mā-Mā
(Morning only. Repeat 3 times.)

Sā-Tu No Pan-Te
(Bow)

The chant is to be followed by offerings from Teachers, Staff, and Students.

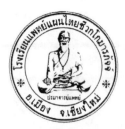

Shivagakomarpaj Lineage "Wai Khru" (Ceremony Honoring the Teacher) Dedicated to Jivaka Komarabhacca, Founder of Thai Medicine

English Translation and Explanation by Tevijjo Yogi

Incantation in honor of Jivaka:
OM. I bow my head in homage to Jivaka.
With compassion for all sentient beings he has brought divine medicine.
Shining bright as the sun and moon, Komarabhacca.
I declare my adoration to the Teacher, the wise one.
May I be free from disease and happy.

Incantation in honor of the Buddha used for generating metta:
Beloved by deities and humans,
Beloved by Brahma, I pay the highest homage.
Beloved by Nagas and heavenly beings,
Of pure faculties, I pay homage.

Untranslated incantation for success in one's practice:
Nā-Mo-Put-Tā-Ya / Nā-Von-Nā-Vean /
Na-Sa-Tit / Na-Sa-Tean / A-Hi-Mā-Mā / Na-Vean-Na-Ve /
Na-Pai-Tang-Vean / Na-Vean-Ma-Ha-Kuu / A-Hi-Ma-Ma /
Pi-Young-Ma-Ma / Nā-Mo-Put-Tā-Ya

Incantation for pacifying the Four Elements:
Na-Ma-Pa-Ta, Honor to the Buddha!

Incantation for healing:
May disease and illness be utterly pacified!

Incantation for bringing good luck:
We invite great prosperity!

Closing incantation:
Well said!

1.

The Classic Thai Massage Routine

Overview of the Classic Routine

1. Opening Prayer

FLUSH TOWARD NAVEL

FEET AND LEG LINES SERIES

2. Walking Palm Press
3. Thumb Press the Feet
4. Thumb Press the Bottom of the Foot, and Thumb Circle the Top of the Foot
5. Pull Each Toe to Crack Knuckles
6. Stretching the Foot
7. Ankle Rotation
   Repeat Steps **3-7** for the other foot
8. Stretching the Feet and Ankles
9. Palm Pressing Both Legs
10. Stretch Inside of Leg
11. Palm Press Inside of Leg
12. Thumb Press Inside Sen of the Leg
    Finish the A-B-C-B-A Pattern by Repeating Palm Press and Stretch
13. Stretch Outside of Same Leg
14. Palm Press Outside of Leg
15. Thumb Press Outside Sen of the Leg
    Finish the A-B-C-B-A Pattern by Repeating Palm Press and Stretch
    Repeat Steps **10-15** for Other Leg
16. Finish the Legs with a Palm Press and "Opening the Wind Gate"

LEG STRETCH SERIES

17. Figure 4 Walking Palm Press
18. Figure 4 Hip Stretch
19. "Paddleboat" on Line **i3**
20. Finger Press on Line **o1**
21. "Thai Fist" on Lines **i1** and **i2**
22. Leg Traction
23. Shake Leg to Relax
24. Hip Rotation
25. Hip Flexion and Quad Stretch
26. Hamstring Stretch
27. Hip Stretch (Lateral Rotation)
28. Lying Spinal Twist
29. Quadriceps Stretch (Medial Rotation of Hip)
30. Shake Leg to Relax
31. Rotate Hip
32. Hamstring and Calf Stretch
33. Triangle (Abduction of Hip)
34. Cross-Stretch (Adduction of Hips)
35. Shake Leg to Relax
    Repeat Steps **17-35** for Other Leg

HANDS AND ARMS SERIES

36. Thumb Press Hand Points
37. Thumb Circle Back of Hand
38. Stretch Palm & Fingers
39. Pull Each Finger and Crack Knuckles
40. Stretch, Palm Press, and Thumb Press Outer Arm Sen
41. Stretch, Palm Press, and Thumb Press Inner Arm Sen
42. Palm Press and Opening the Wind Gate
43. Rotate Wrist
44. Rotate Elbow
45. Rotate Shoulder
46. Pull Arm to Stretch
47. Medial Arm Pull
48. Stretch the Triceps
49. Palm Press Arm Above Head
50. Shake Arm to Relax
    Repeat Steps **36-50** for Opposite Side

ABDOMINAL SERIES

51. Finger Press Below Clavicles
52. Finger Circle Rib Cage
53. Thumb Press or Finger Press in the Intercostal Spaces
54. Palm Circle and Press on Sternum
55. Palm Circles on Abdomen

56. Palm Press Abdomen
57. Thumb Press Around Navel
58. Finger Press Psoas
59. Back Lift
60. Rock Hips to Relax

FULL-BODY STRETCHES

61. Gentle Back Stretch
62. Lower Hamstring Stretch
63. Upper Hamstring Stretch
64. Pigeon Pose
Repeat **62-64** for the other leg
65. The Plow
66. Butterfly
67. Double Leg Pull-Up
68. Cross-Legged Pull-Up
69. Forward Bend with Crossed Legs
70. Bound Angle Pose
71. Forward Bend with Straight Legs
72. Forward Bend with Wide-Angle Legs
73. "Motorcycle" Back Stretch
74. Fish Pose
75. Seated Spinal Twist
76. Back Lift
77. Thai Chop on Back

OPTIONAL THERAPY ROUTINE

FLUSH TOWARD CROWN

BACK SERIES

78. Knee Press Feet
79. Thumb Press Foot Points
80. Stretch Legs
81. Palm Press Legs
82. Thumb Press Along Line **i3**
Finish the A-B-C-B-A Pattern by Repeating Palm Press and Stretch
83. Forearm Roll the Hamstrings
84. Elbow Press Along Line **i3**
85. Rotate Ankle
86. Calf Stretch
87. Knee Flexion

Repeat Steps **83-87** for the Other Side
88. Thumb Press Hip Points
89. Finger Press or Elbow Press Gluteal Muscles
90. Palm Circle Sacrum
91. Stretch Back
92. Palm Press Back
93. Thumb Press Sen of the Back
Finish A-B-C-B-A Pattern by Repeating Palm Press and Stretch
94. Palm Circle Rib Cage
95. Pull Trapezius Muscles
96. Shoulder Mobilization
97. Press Under Scapula
98. Cobra
99. Single-Leg Locust

HEAD, NECK, AND FACE SERIES

100. Thumb Press Under Clavicles
101. Gently Stretch Neck by Pressing on Shoulders
102. Ear Massage
Repeat **101-102** for the Other Side
103. Finger Press Along Trapezius and Neck
104. Base of Skull and Back of Head
105. Forehead and Chin Lines
106. Scrub Scalp with "Shampooing" Motion

FULL-BODY FLUSH & FINAL METTA

107. Create a Vacuum with the Ears
108. Finish with a Meditation of Thanksgiving and Healing

1. Opening Prayer

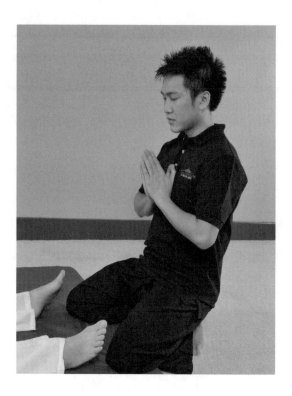

Feet and Leg Lines Series

2. Walking Palm Press

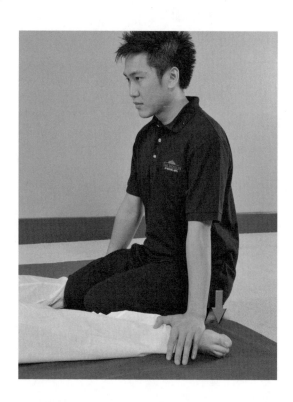

3. Thumb Press the Feet

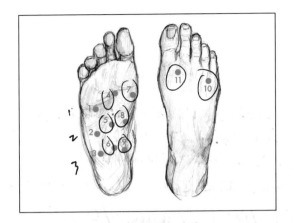

* Hombres pie derecho
* Mujeres pie izquierdo.
* Poner el pie sobre mi pierna

- Despues de los puntos de presion.
- Otra vez los puntos y Jalar
- Coda dedo presecito.
- Siempre del Talou. Por arriba
- Luego un Stretch very nice

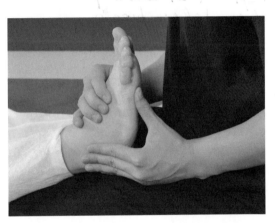

**4. Thumb Press the Bottom of the Foot,
and Thumb Circle the Top of the Foot**

4 & 5 Conclusive.

- En esta figura hacemos 3
circulos y todo se
Mueve en circulos.

- Se Jala cada dedo fuerte

- al final Stречh fuerte
o sea Jalar fuerte.

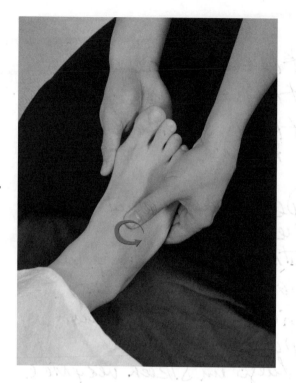

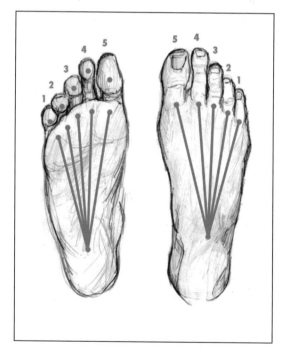

5. Pull Each Toe to Crack Knuckles

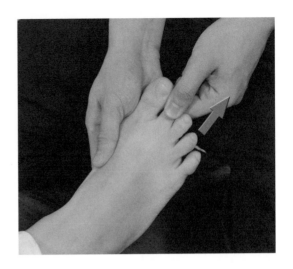

6. Stretching the Foot

✳ Mover el cuerpo cuando siéamos el autle. Tis veces auebos lados.

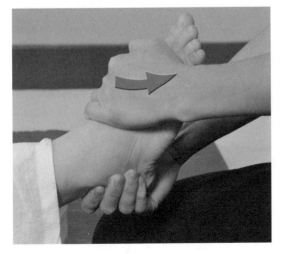
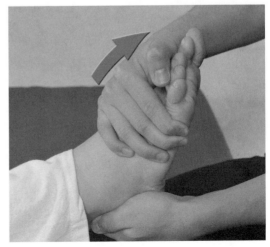

(10 minutes!)

7. Ankle Rotation
Repeat Steps **3–7** for the other foot

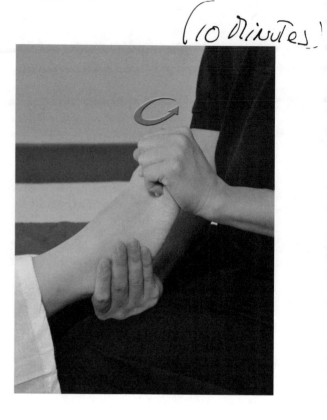

Legs — 30 minutes

8. Stretching the Feet and Ankles

Presionar hacia el suelo #1

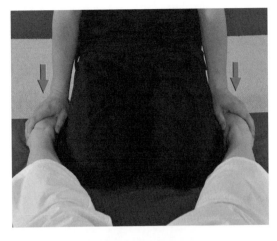

Empujar los dedos hacia la cabeza. #2

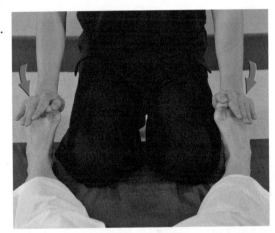

Empujar los dedos inward. #3
Shake the legs nicely.

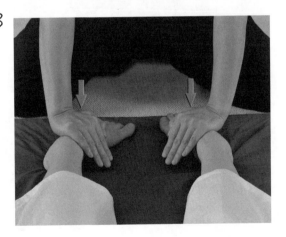

9. Palm Pressing Both Legs

Start left.

las rodillas 3 Times

Palm walk toward Hips.

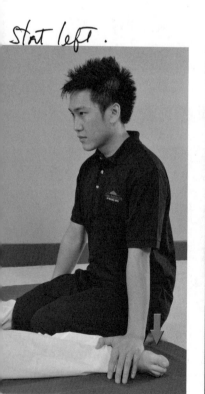
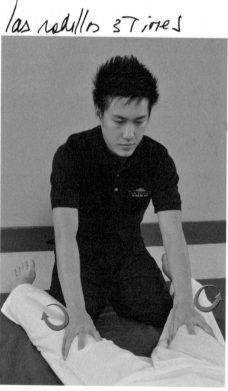
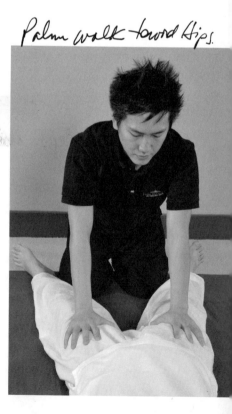

1/20/2013

entan dentro de los 2 piernos osea en medio. de

10. Stretch Inside of Leg

both hands equal pressure.

A. ... ~~Palm pressure~~ . Stretch
B. ... Palm
C. .. sen work . (2 veces)
B. ... Palm
A. ..... Stretch

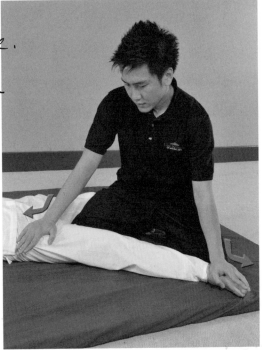

11. Palm Press Inside of Leg

Start from the ankle.
Rocking slowly. all the way up
and back down

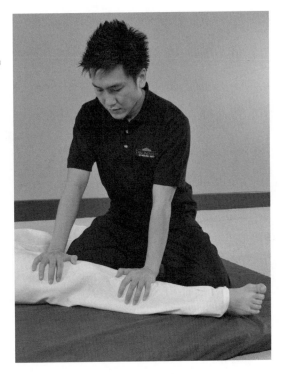

12. Thumb Press Inside *Sen* of the Leg

A — Stretch

B — ~~Palm press~~ Palm press.

C — SEN work (2 lees)

B — Palm Press

A — Stretch.

La Segunda linea de Sen
los dedos van dentro del
Muslo.

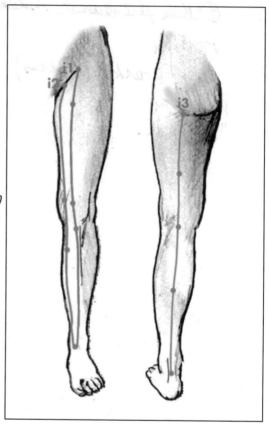

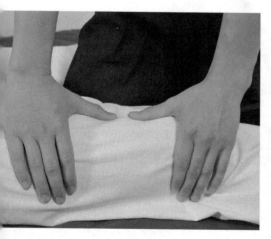
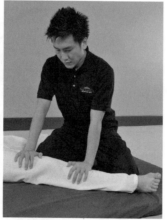
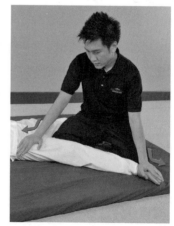

Finish by Repeating Palm Press (Step **11**) and Stretch (Step **10**) to Complete the A-B-C-B-A Pattern.

sentarse fuera de las piernas y traer el acaba

13. Stretch Outside of Same Leg

Soft

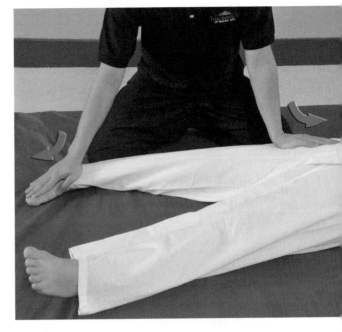

14. Palm Press Outside of Leg

Back and forth

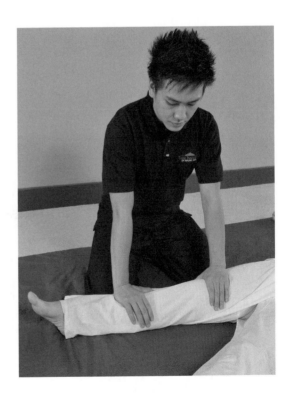

15. Thumb Press Outside *Sen* of the Leg

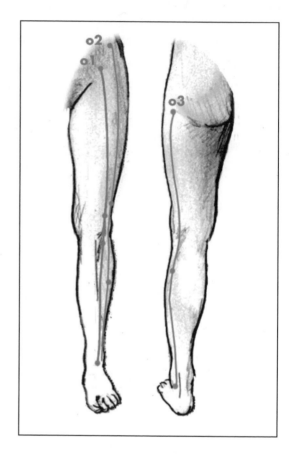

Do the Senp work.

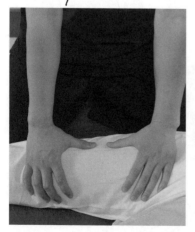
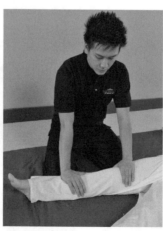
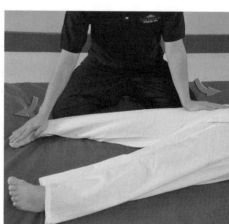

Finish by repeating Palm Press & Stretch to complete the A-B-C-B-A Pattern.
Repeat Steps **10-15** for other Leg.

Abrir los dos puernos y Meterse adentro, Compresiones al final.

22

VARIATION: **Alternate Position for Leg Lines**

16. **Finish the Legs with a Palm Press** and
    "Opening the Wind Gate"

Do Palm press Compresions.

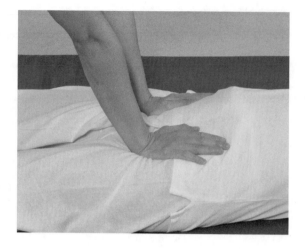

VARIATION: **Opening the Wind Gate in the Legs**

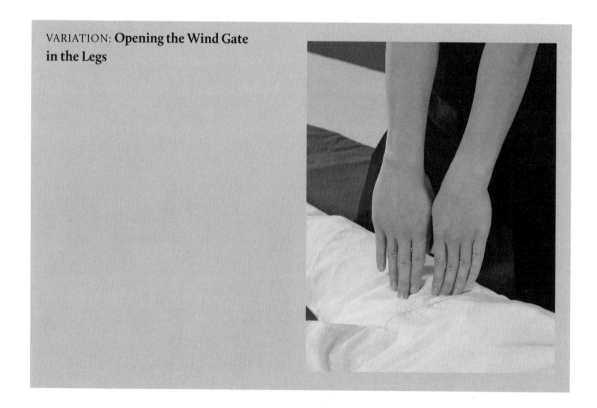

Male Right leg
female left leg.

Sentense afueen
del 4

Leg Stretch Series

17. Figure 4 Walking Palm Press

- Figure 4 — No use pillow.
- Palm press.
- all the way to the knee.

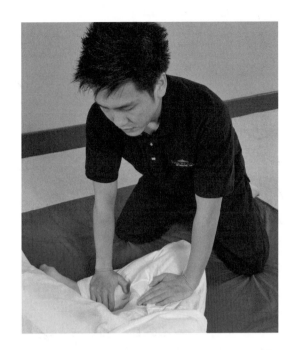

18. Figure Four Hip Stretch

- so perpendicular to the knee.
- Nice palm press to the legs.
  all the way to the knees
- Do once.

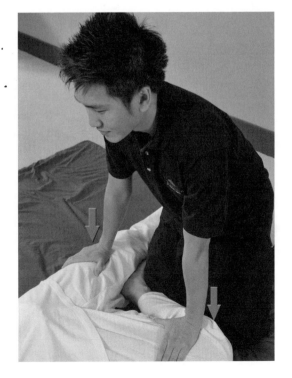

19. "Paddleboat" on Line i3

Open the leg nice.
Leave the other leg nice & straight
Sole of the feet in the hamshrings
Grave the ankle.
Walk around the SEN.
Pull the ankle to create tension
Pull the leg over and hug the foot
Reach over his guards.
Lean back. & Move up.
Back & Forth
Stay Position.
Tish Fist around the guards.
Back & Forth

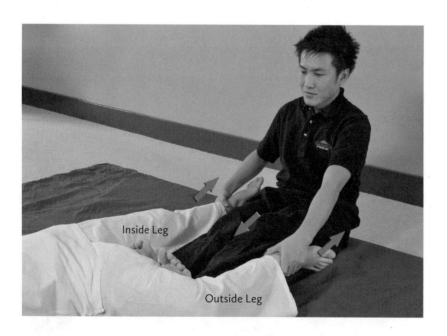

Inside Leg

Outside Leg

20. Finger Press on Line o1

La pierna encima de
Mis pies.
Jalar el muslo.
golpear con los puños

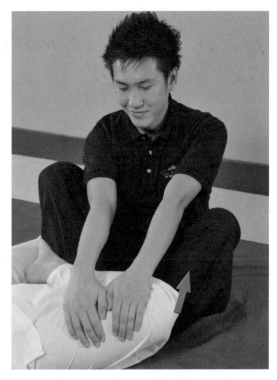

21. Thai Fist on Lines i1 and i2

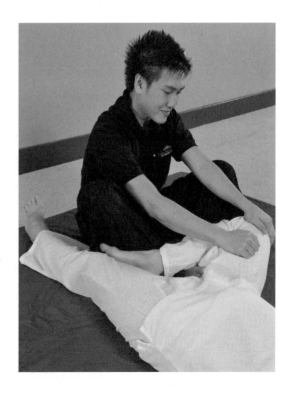

22. Leg Traction

Meter el pie en el muslo
Jalar hacia Mi

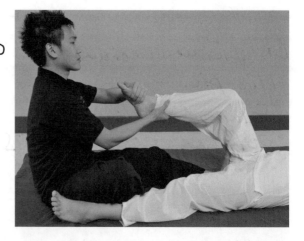

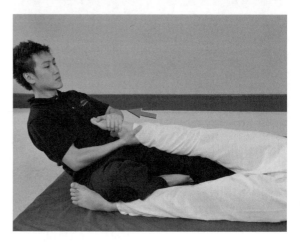

23. Shake Leg to Relax

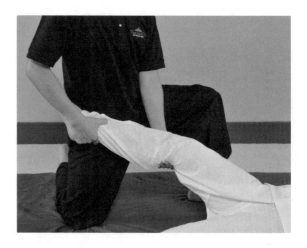

24. Hip Rotation

♀ 80/20   RoTar la
cadera
3 vees
cada
lado.
Mover Mi
CueRpo.

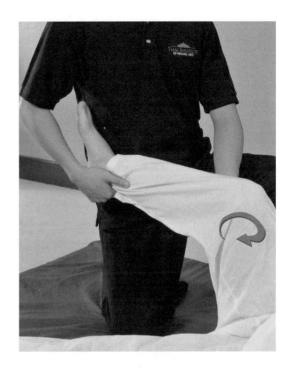

25. Hip Flexion & Quad Stretch

EMpusar la pierna
Hacia El Pecho

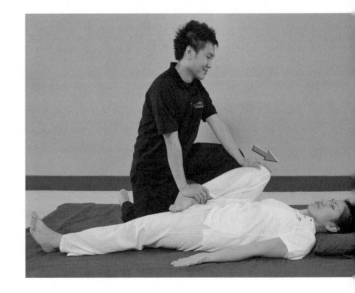

VARIATION: **Pigeon Pose**

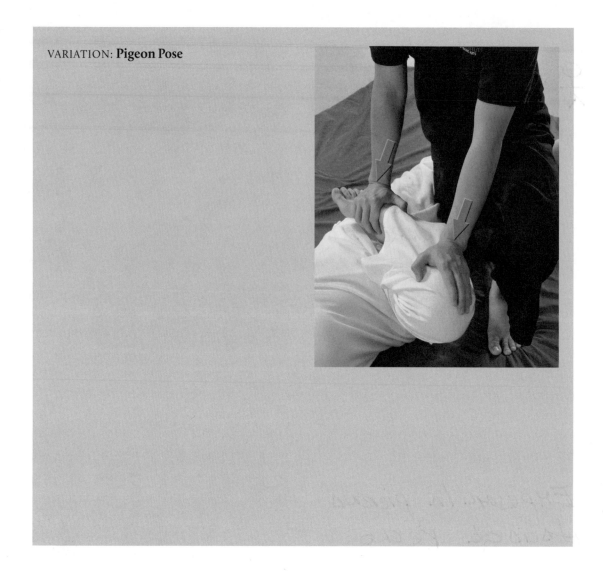

26. Hamstring Stretch

Empusar La pierna y mi mano en el otro muslo.

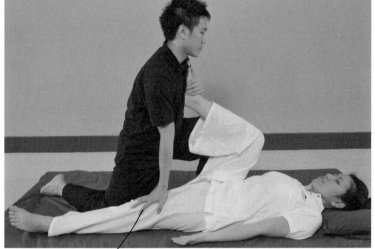

Correct Alignment & be careful with the fingers, make sure to have the hands in the direction of the foot.

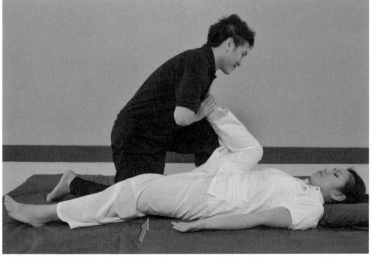

Incorrect Alignment

27. Hip Stretch (Lateral Rotation)

— the foot in the Hip pocket .
— hand on the guards .
— Knee towards the arm pit

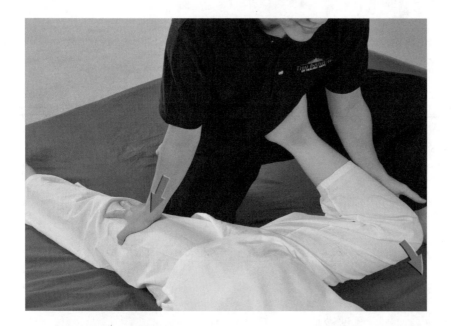

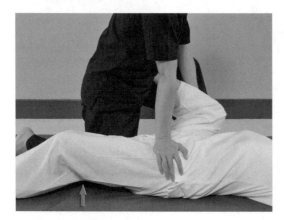

Incorrect Alignment

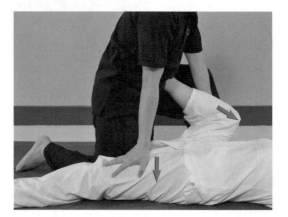

Correct Alignment

28. Lying Spinal Twist

♀ 80/20. llevar la pierna
al otro lado.
y luego
EMPUJAR LA
PIERNA
AGARRANDO la
Codera.
Sacudir LA
PIERNA.
Mecer La PIERNA ~~3~~
veces aCada LADO

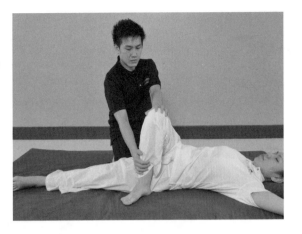

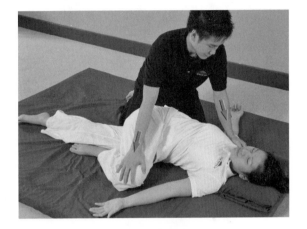

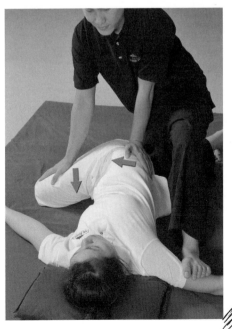

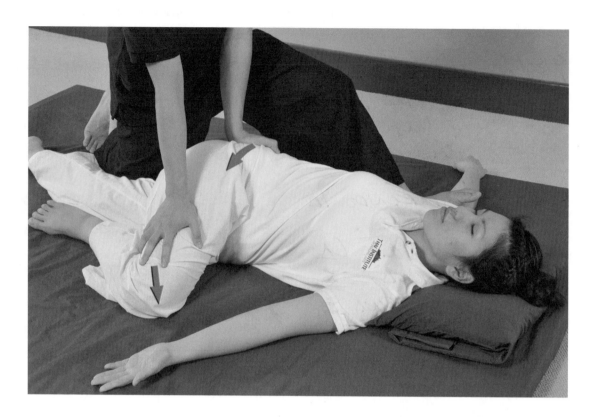

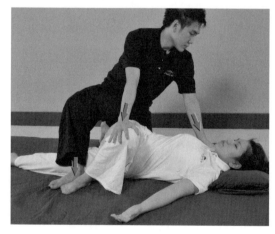

29. Quadriceps Stretch
   (Medial Rotation of Hip)

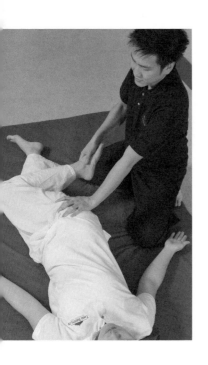 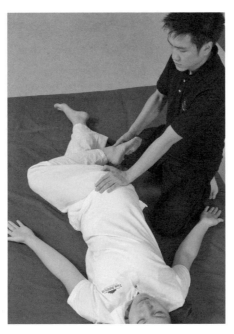 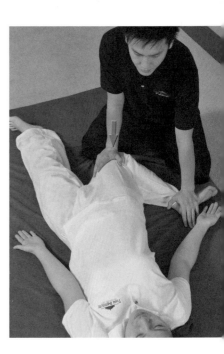

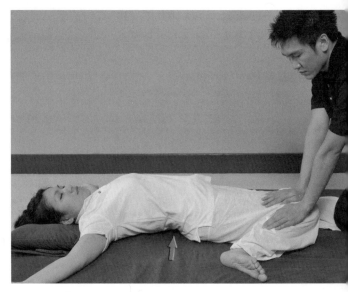

Incorrect Alignment

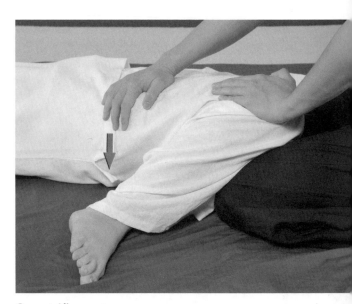

Correct Alignment

VARIATION: **Finger Press Iliopsoas**

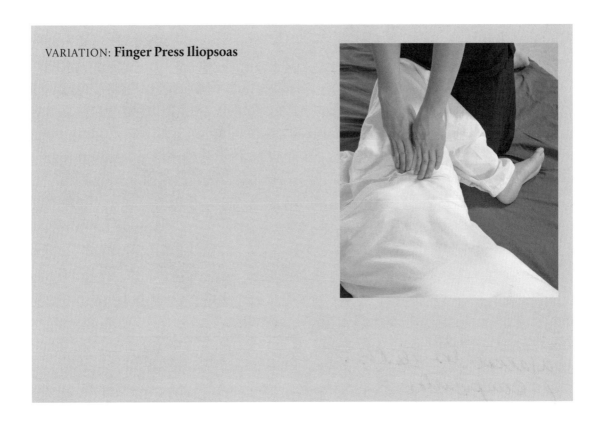

30. Shake Leg to Relax
Same as step **23**.

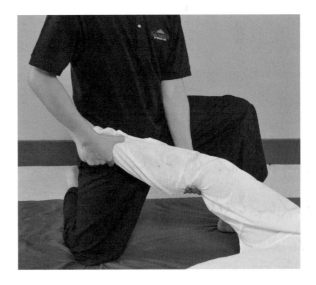

31. Rotate Hip

palm of an hand in te Hell

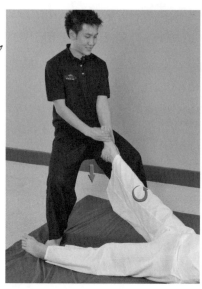

32. Hamstring and Calf Stretch

agarran los dedos.
y empujartos

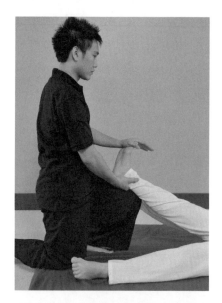

agarran el pié
PResionan el Muslo

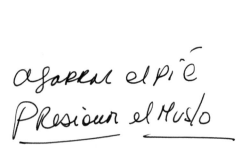

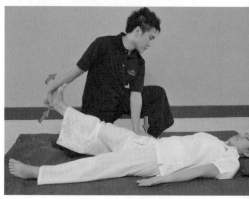

elevar la pierna. Sobre Mi Hombro
y empujar el otro Muslo
Mis dedos en dirección
del pié.

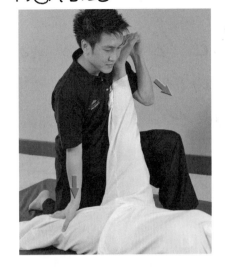

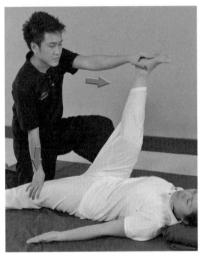

be Mindful with your foot.
Sobre el Muslo.

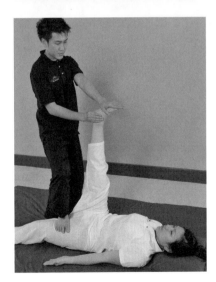

33. Triangle (Abduction of Hip)

Abrir La pierna hacia fuera.
PRESIONAR.
Golpear.

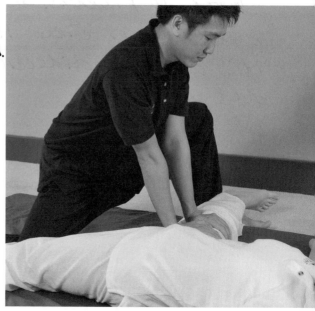

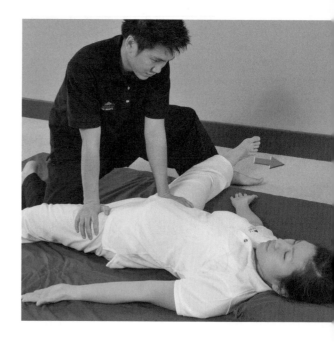

34. Cross-Stretch (Adduction of Hips)

Estinar La piernas luego solpecitos .

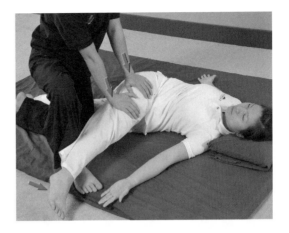

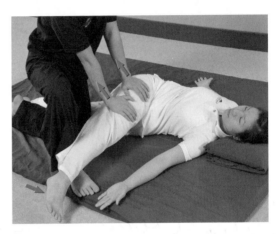

35. Shake Leg to Relax It

*TERMINAR CON COMPRESIÓNES.
De ida y vuelta .*

Repeat Steps **17-35** for other leg.
Finish leg routine by palm pressing both legs.
(**S**ee Step **9**.)

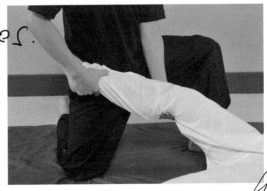

*Terminamos en la Guaira de Morts
Classes .*

Tarde del Marks.
BRMS — 21 Minutes

Hands and Arms Series

36. Thumb Press Hand Points

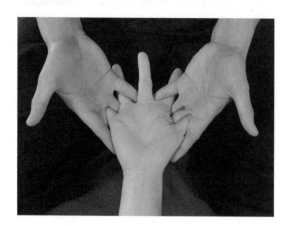
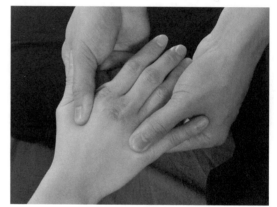

Cada ½ gm pusieran
se jala la Mano cuando termina.

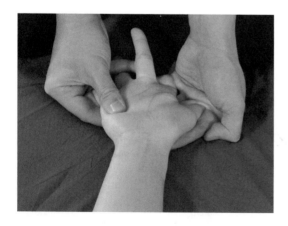
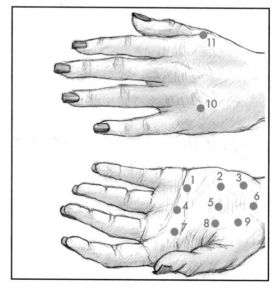

37. Thumb Circle Back of Hand

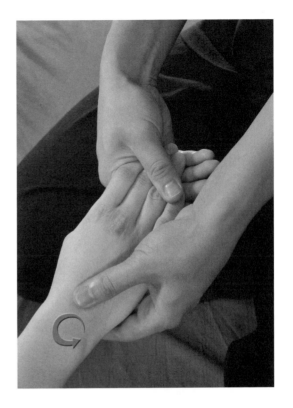

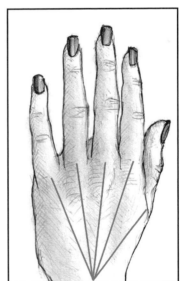

38.   Stretch Palm and Fingers

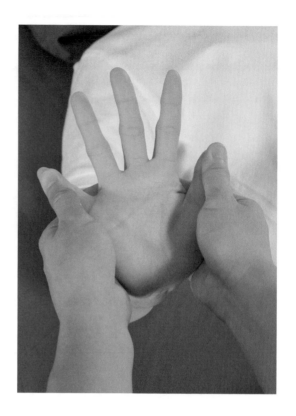

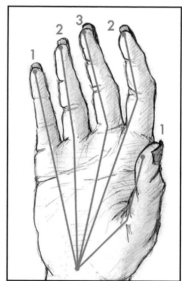

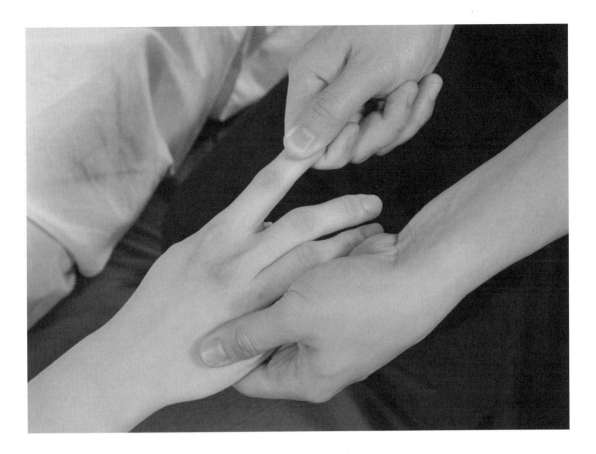

39.   Pull Each Finger and Crack Knuckles

40. Stretch, Palm Press, and Thumb Press Outer Arm *Sen*

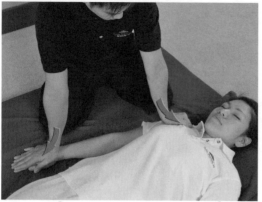 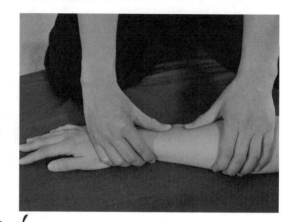

a— Strech. lean forward.
b— Palm press.
c— Sen Work.
b— Palm press.
a— Strech.

Finish the A-B-C-B-A pattern by repeating the palm press and stretch.

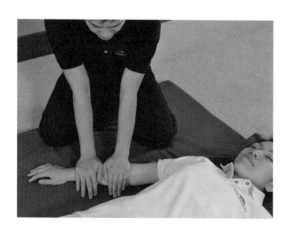 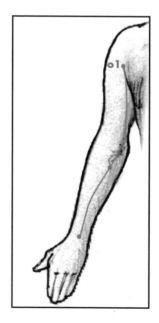

41. Stretch, Palm Press, and Thumb Press Inner Arm *Sen*

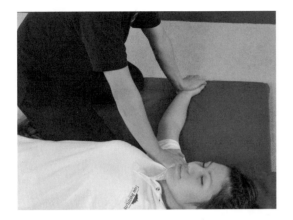
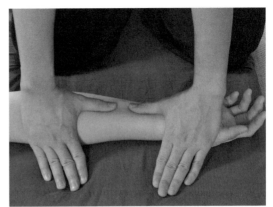

Finish the A-B-C-B-A pattern by repeating the palm press and stretch.

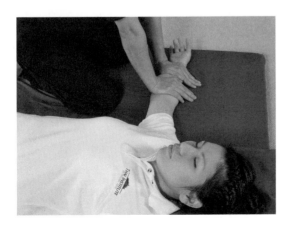
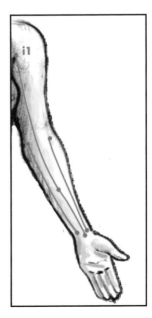

42. Opening the Wind Gate

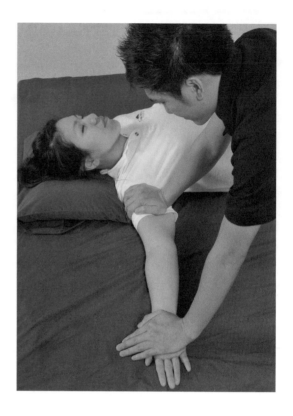

43. Rotate Wrist

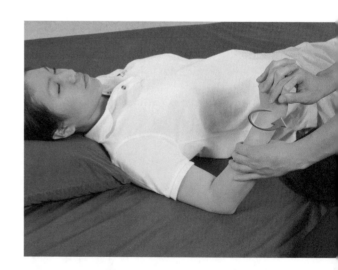

44. Rotate Elbow

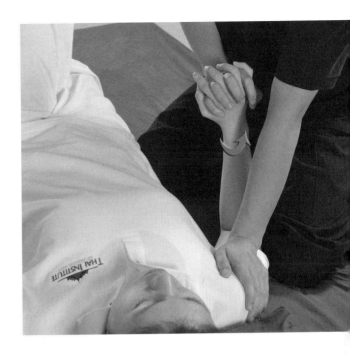

45. Rotate Shoulder

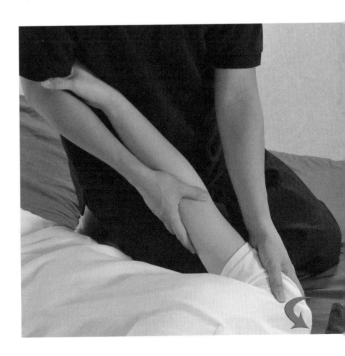

46. Pull Arm to Stretch

Streches ①

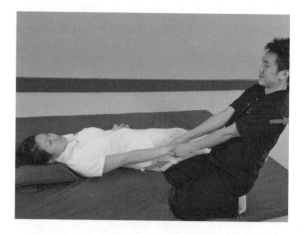

Streels (2)

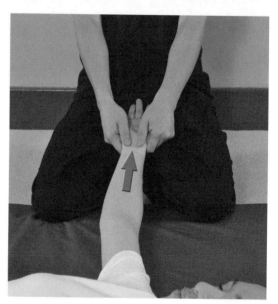

Streeches (3).
TUPAC AMARU.

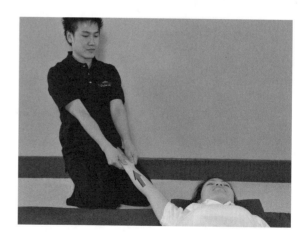

47. Medial Arm Pull

Step over.
mismo en la Rodilla.
lean forward.
Variation:
Caminar al otro lado
& luego hacer Stretch.

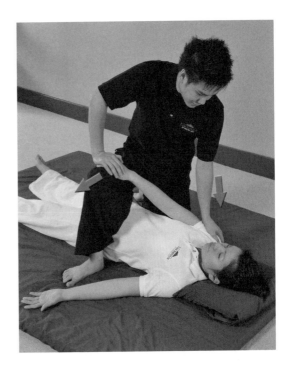

48. Stretch the triceps

Strech al lado de la oreja A.
pecno la mano B.
palm to Palm. C.
Finger Tracing the feet. B.
Stech poner la mano D.
en la codera...
press the arm.
presiona con el dedo gorlo.
palm press.
Twisted with the Stech.

attention!

poner el brazo sobre la cabeza.
Hacerlo despacio no hacer
doler al cliente.

usar el pillar
press compresion
lerejo strke

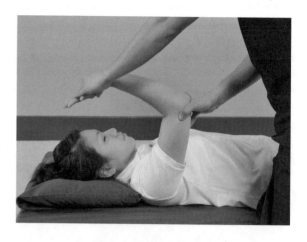

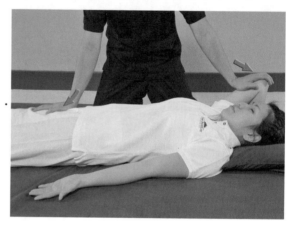

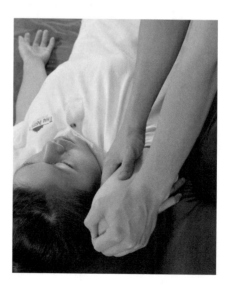

Finish the A-B-C-B-A pattern by repeating
the palm press and stretch.

VARIATION: **For Less Flexible Clients**

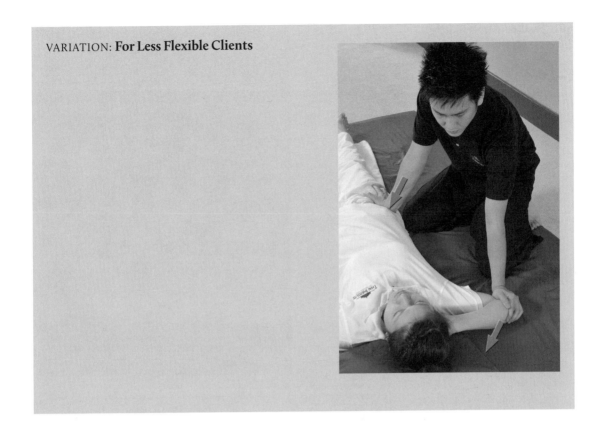

49. Palm Press Arm Above Head

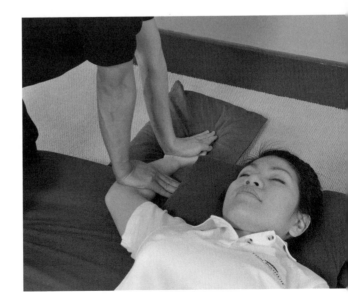

50. Shake Arm to Relax
Repeat Steps **36-50** for opposite side.

Sacudir

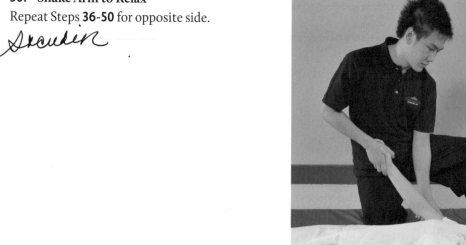

Abdominal Series

51. Finger Press Below Clavicles

de afuera hacia dentro

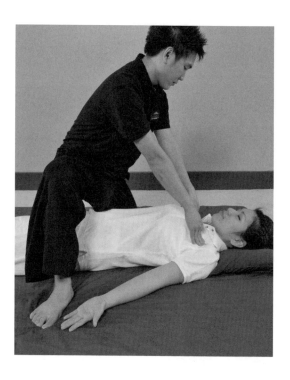

52. Finger Circle Rib Cage

los movimitos hacia arriba.

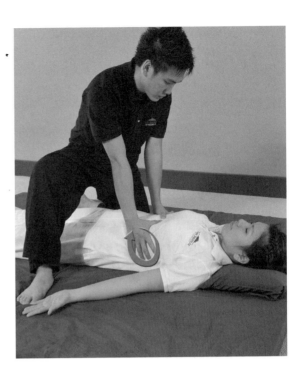

53. Thumb Press or Finger Press in the Intercostal Spaces

*hacer coda una de las
Costillas con presión
de los dedos.
Ø empezar desde arriba
Test: hacer una az colando*

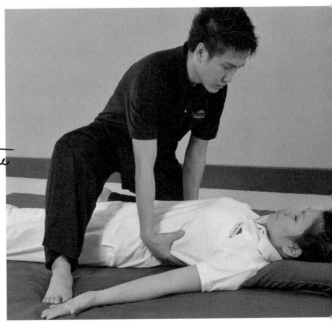

54. Palm Circle and Press on Sternum

① *light presure*.

✳ mano sobre la mano.
rotation.
3 rec cada lodo.
presione suave.

✳ female client
usar sus manos
poner una mano sobre
la otra y hacer to
mismo ①

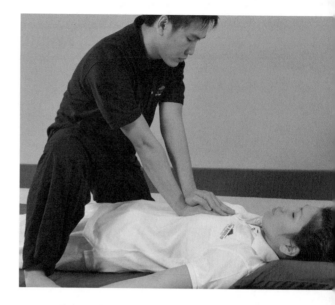

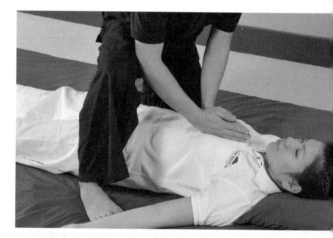

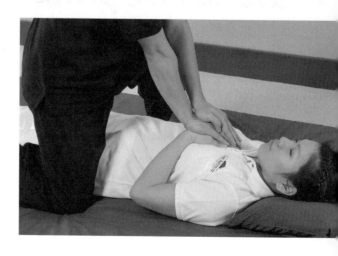

55. Palm Circles on Abdomen *Skip .*

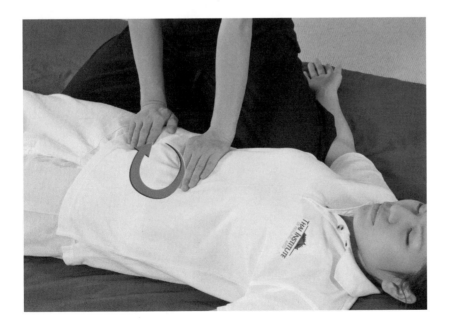

56. Palm Press Abdomen *Skip*

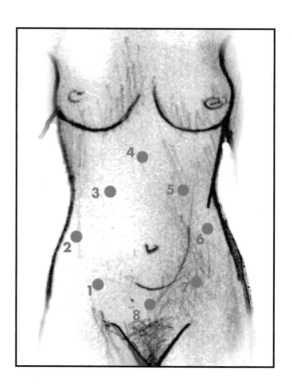

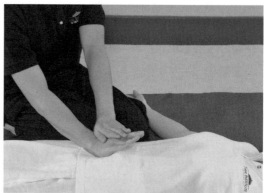

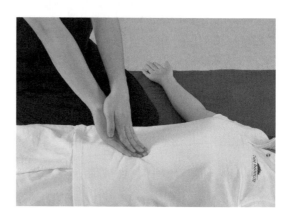

Skip

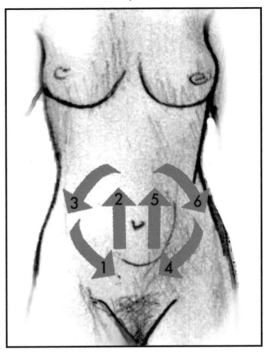

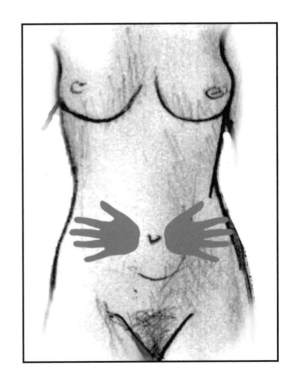

57.   Thumb Press Around Navel

Rock the Hip. to 61.
& Lift the Hip. (Legs).
bend the knees.
Put his knees right on my
knee.
and gentle press to stretch
his back.

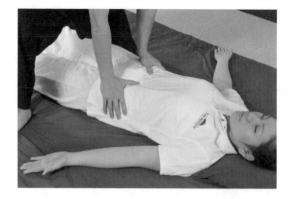

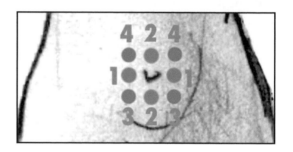

58.   Finger Press Psoas

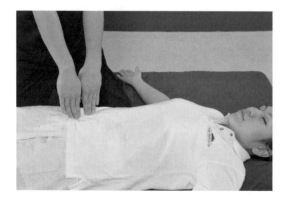

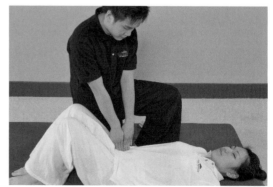

59. Back Lift

Usar los dedos .
Hacerlo 3 secs .
Calentar .

ask for deep breath
levantar el cuerpo.

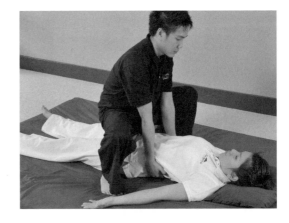

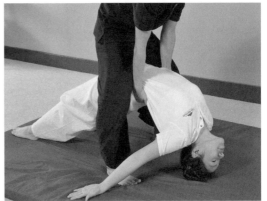

fin de Martes por la tarde.

60. Rock Hips to Relax

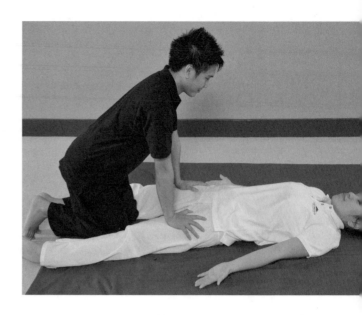

Full-Body Stretches (3 Things each leg)

61. Gentle Back Stretch

① they

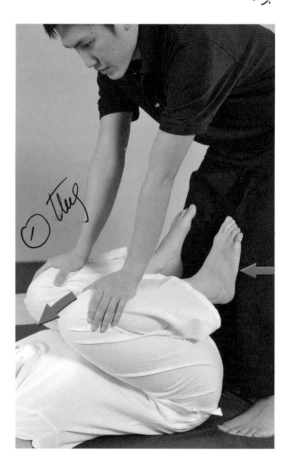

Wed - Morning Day 3rd

62. Lower Hamstring Stretch

Forearm rolls.

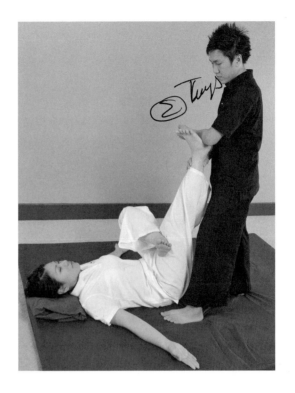

63. Upper Hamstring Stretch

80/20.

— outside hand.
— press de foot
— otten hand in the slut

— Let the leg rest on my lap.

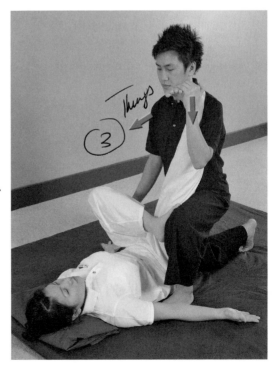

VARIATION: **For Hamstring Stretch**

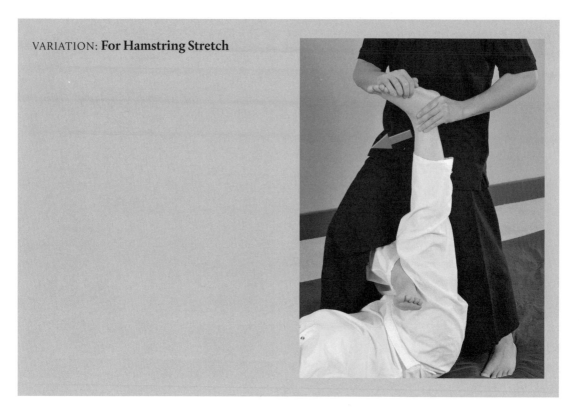

DAY 3.

64. Pigeon Pose
Repeat **62-64** for the other leg.

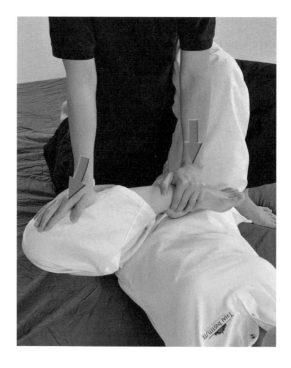

65. The Plow

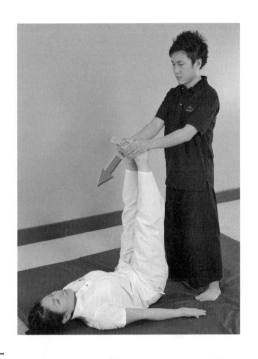

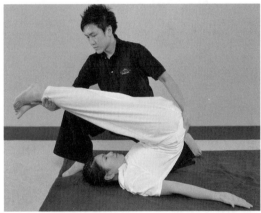

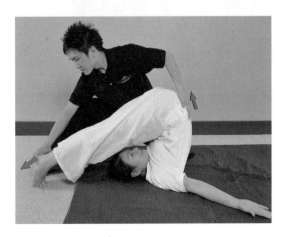

♀ 80/20.
Step over the arm.
Take outside arm – (hand).
Come around.
Hold the heels.
the ~~other~~ hand place
on the Sacrum.
Hold the Sacrum
~~Hold the~~ Heel.
Hold the legs around
then my belly.

Skip. X

VARIATIONS: **For Less Flexible Clients**

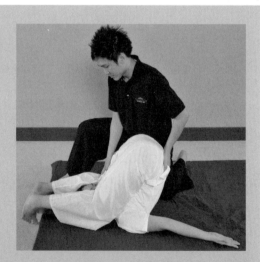

Day 3.

66. Butterfly

— Spread the leg
Toes underneath.
bring the legs
push away
Start bending your knees.
ask the client is okay..
— Step out
Holding the legs
— Keep the legs in my Belly..

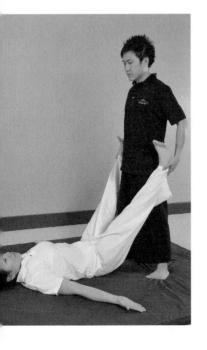
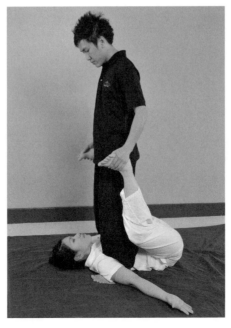
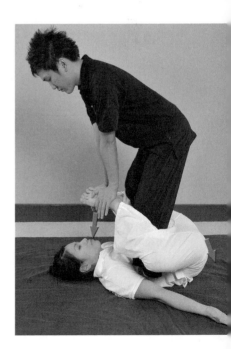

Day 3

67. **Double Leg Pull-Up**

- Legs en su belly.
- Palms up (como pidiendo algo)
- agarrar los 2 forearms.
- estar derecho.
- asir el pecho.

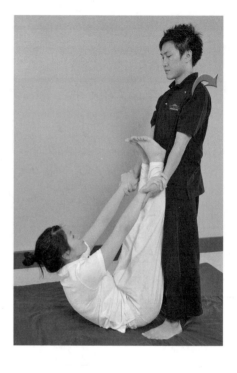

68. **Cross-Legged Pull-Up**

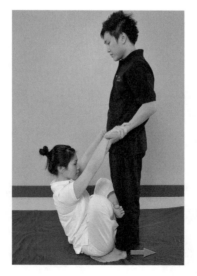 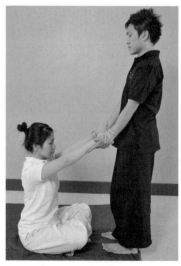

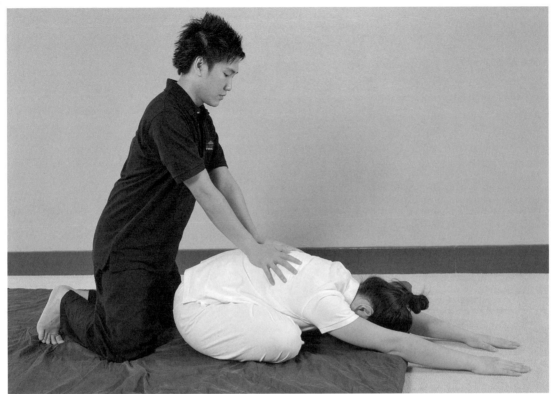

walk around his back.

69. Forward Bend with Crossed Legs

— gentle press — palm press.
— Forearm Rolls.
— bring them back to sit.

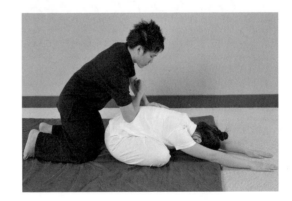

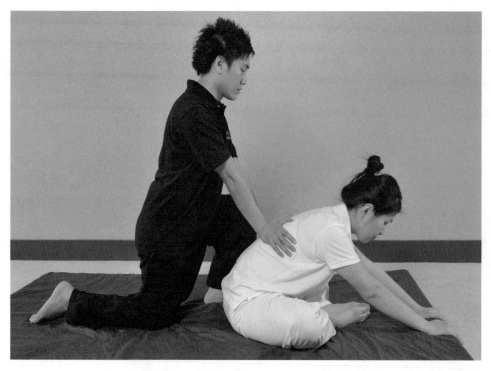

70. Bound-Angle Pose

We have to put their feet together.
Take their hands on the mat.

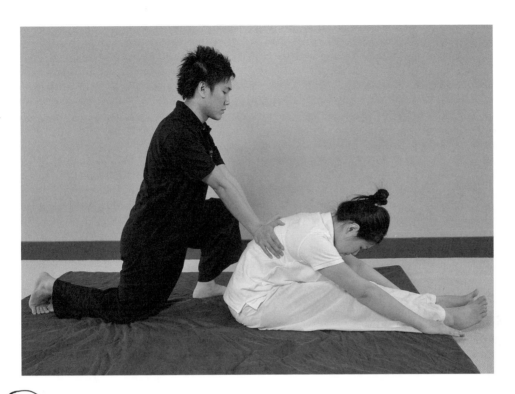

71. **Forward Bend with Straight Legs**

— Palm press
— forearm rolls .
— Hand on the Sacrum.
— Hand on the Shoulder.

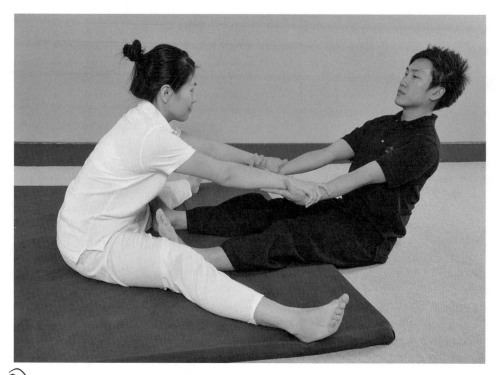

72. Forward Bend with Wide-Angle Legs

— open their legs.
— place my feet under their knees.
— grab their forearm
— then stretch. (depend on each person).
—————
— put their legs together

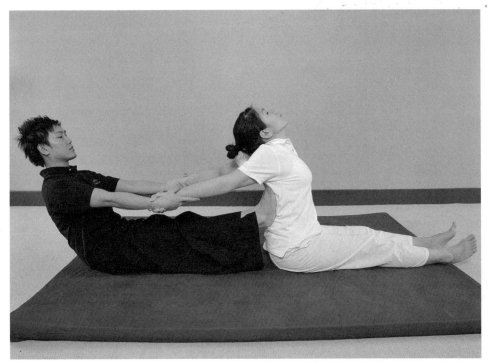

73. "Motorcycle" Back Stretch   (Esto no es bueno para personas con shoulders problemas.)

— ponerse detros del Cliente
— Mis pies en el Sacrum – luego en el Shoulder blades.
— agarrar forearm – (Mis piernos con los rodillos dobladas)
— luego Estirar mis piernas – (Palmas out) afuera. ncia.
— Mirar hacia arriba
— luego release their arms.

— Mis pies en el Sacrum Nuevamente.
— agarrar el pillow.
— ponerlo en el Sacrum
— agarrar los hombros.
— Jalar.
— La Cabeza en Mi Mano izquierda.
— luego los dos Manos en la cabeza sostener la cabeza
— Clientes con los manos o palmas hacia arriba.
— luego Mi mano derecha empujar
— Mano izquierda sostiene la cabeza
— Regresar los 2 al mismo tiempo
— Mis rodillos siempre estan dobladas.

Day 3.
all break 14 Minutes.

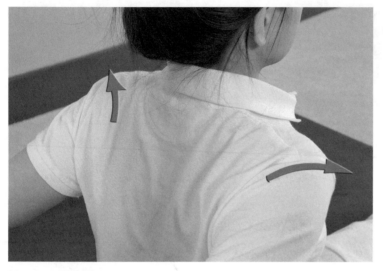

Incorrect Alignment

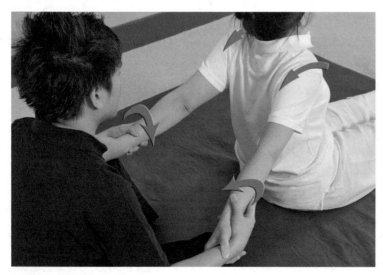

Correct Alignment

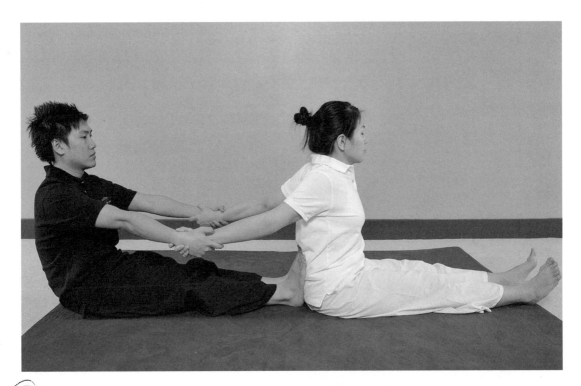

74. Fish Pose

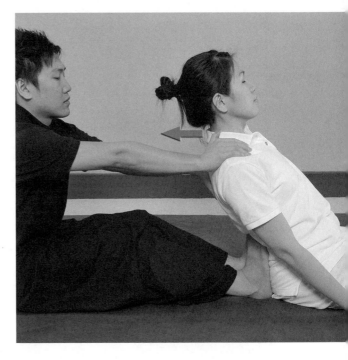

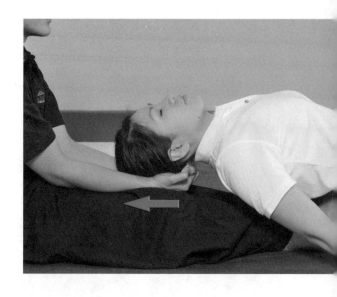

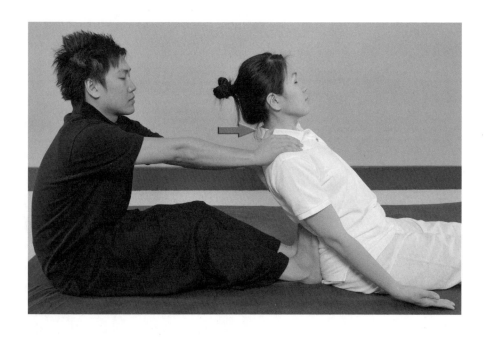

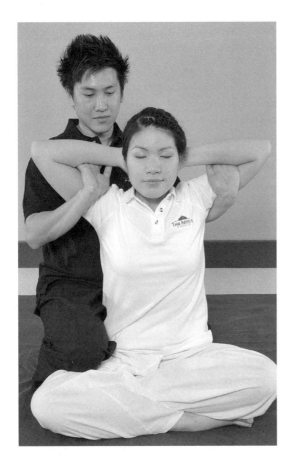 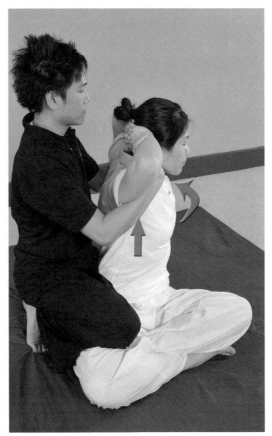

75. **Seated Spinal Twist**

Day 3

Best for "us"

VARIATION: **For Increased Leverage**

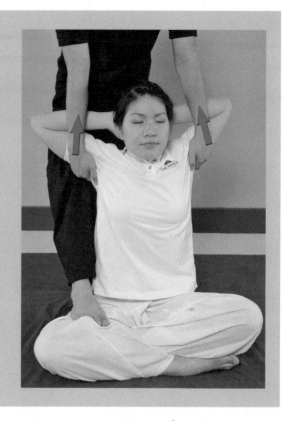

— Agarrar al cliente debajo de los hombros.
Cerca a la axila.
— Jalar hacia arriba
— Luego Twist — 3 veces. los dos lados

76. **Back Lift**

— Suben los brazos.
— agarrarlos Muñecas.
— Los dos al mismo Tiempo
— Doslar mis Rodillas.
— poner sus brazos a bajo.

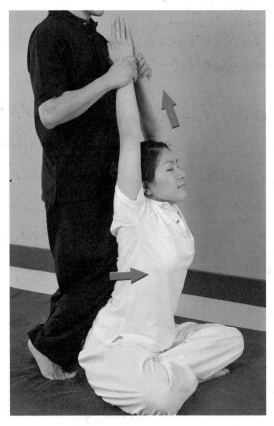

77. **Thai Chop on Back**

— Sus Manos en sus Rodillas.
— luego Thai Chop.
— Sobre los hombros.

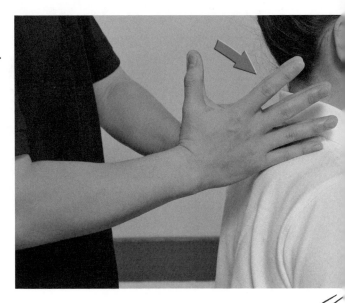

Day 4   1/24/2013.

Boca abajo.

* poner pillow en la casa.   **Back Series**
* Poner una toalla.

78. Knee Press Feet

* los pies Tienen que estar Mirando bien adentro.

* Knee on the Ball — La rodilla en la planta del pie.

* agarrar los talons, Mi cuerpo tiene que estar derecho.

* Otra Manera: Mi pie Cruzado luego Caminar.

* También usar los Talons, luego Balancear Suovemente

```
— a
— b
— c
— b
— a
```

Caminar sobre la planta de los pies

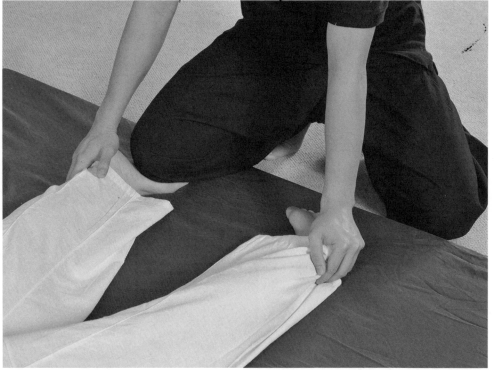

79. Thumb Press Foot Points

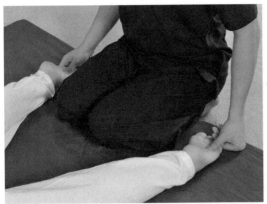
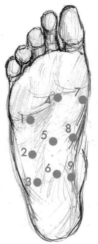
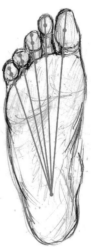

Otra vez presionar, mover el cuerpo de adelante hacia atrás suavemente.

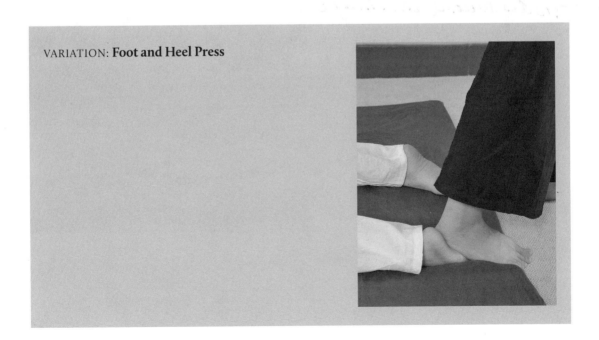

VARIATION: **Foot and Heel Press**

80. Stretch Legs

- Strech las piernas Los 2 el mismo Tiempo.
- luego pump press.
- all the way hasta las gluteos
- Rocking back & forth.
- Sen line
- Start Aquiles tendon (arriba).
- Hacer los 2 piernas el mismo Tiempo.
-

a
b
c
h
g

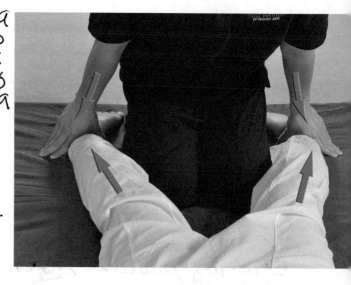

81. Palm Press Legs

- Los dos manos al mismo tiempo.

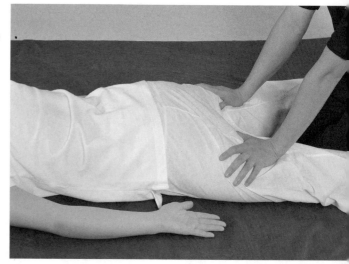

Day 4.

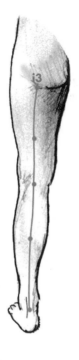

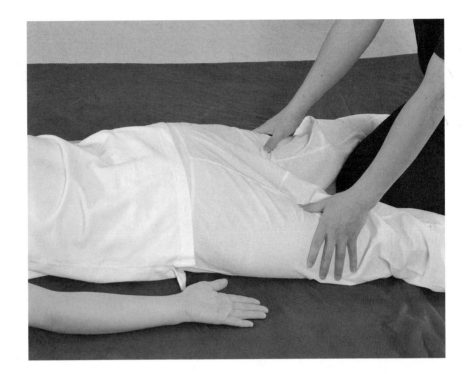

82. **Thumb Press Along Line i3**

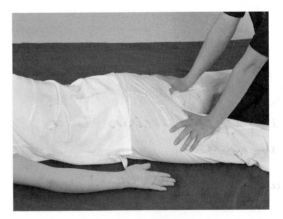

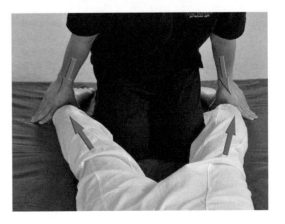

Finish the A-B-C-B-A pattern by repeating
the palm press and stretch.

Day 4.

83. Forearm Roll the Hamstrings

- Forearm Solo en los Muslos.
- Luego usar el Codo Soft
- Cerrar el Codo luego abirlo.

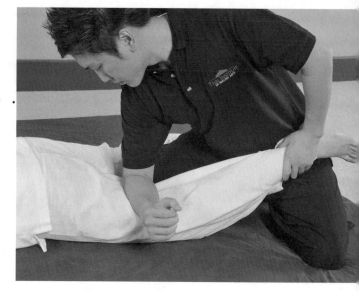

84. Elbow Press Along i3

Codo llevar locales gluteos
suavemente.
Tecnica Forearm Rolls.

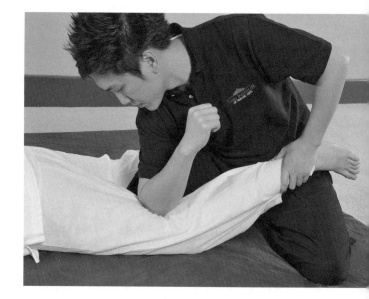

85. Rotate Ankle agarrar los dedos.

5 veces al derecho
5 ✓ a la izquierda.
Moverse con el cuerpo.

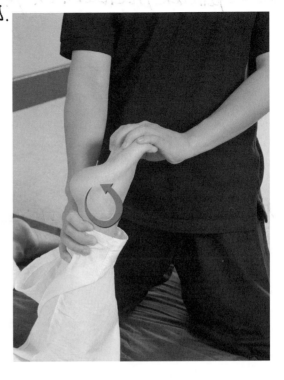

86. Calf Stretch

- Presionar con el codo.
en la planta del pie.
- Presionar con el codo.
y presionar

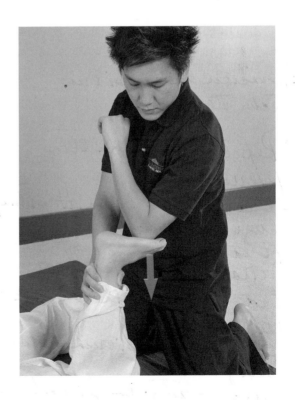

Del 4.
Usa
Mano izquierda presionen la pieren.

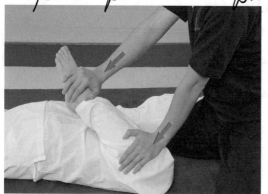

La Mano derecha alzar la pierna.

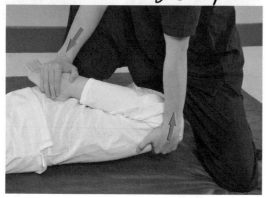

VARIATIONS:

Skip.

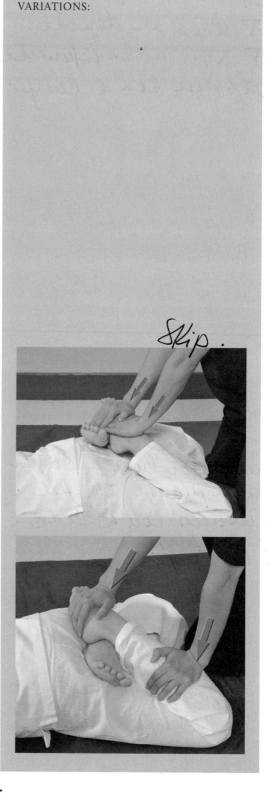

87. Knee Flexion
Repeat Steps **83-87** for the other side.

Elevación de la pieren
Strech the Psoas.

#) Repetin todo el la otra
pierna:
Forearm en la pierna Hamstrings
luego soft Codo.
Forearm.
Rotación de los tobillos.
Codo en la planta del pie.
luego:
presiono la pierna en cenlen
del glúteo.
luego levantar la pierna para
estirar el Psoas.

86

(88.) Thumb Press Hip Points

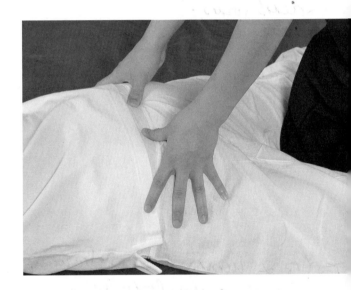

Con los palmos asientes
usar el dedo gordo.
presiouen 1 - 2 - 3
en forma de Triangulo.

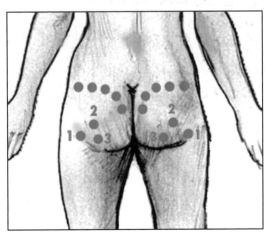

89. Finger Press or Elbow Press
Gluteal Muscles

* Empezar en los bordes.
* Usar los dedos gordos.
  Seguir los bordes del
  Sacrum.
  Luego regresar hacia arriba.

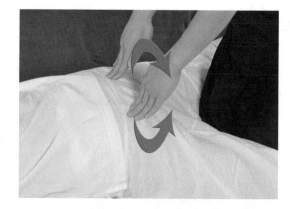

* usar las dos manos.
  hacer los 2 glúteos al mismo
  tiempo.
  —dedos gordos.
  —Todos los dedos.
  —Fist.
  —Codos

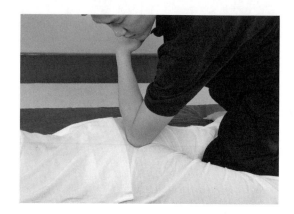

90. Palm Circle Sacrum

* Los 2 manos sobre el Sacrum.
  5 veces a un lado en
  círculos
    Luego 5 veces al Otro lado.
* Puede ser despacio
  o puede ser más rápido.

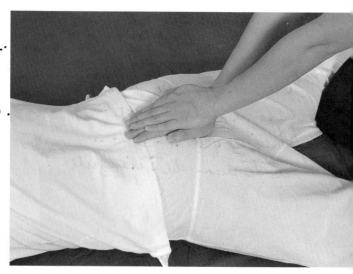

91   Stretch Back

9 —
5 —
C —
6 —
9 —

.80/20 la mano derecha
en la escapula
la mano izquierda
sobre el Riñón
la mano izquierda
es la que trabaja
presiona —

* Hacer las dos escapulas.
* Luego Compresiones.
  alrededor de la Columna.
* .

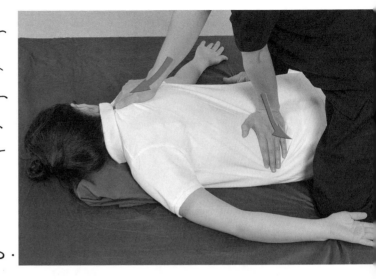

92.   Palm Press Back

Las palmas de arriba
hacia abajo 2 veces.
luego tira el aire
hacia afuera.

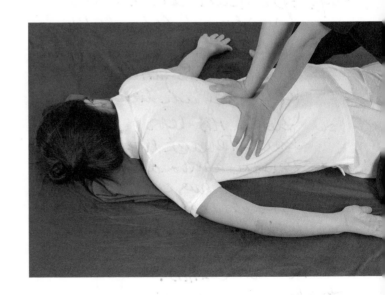

Day 4

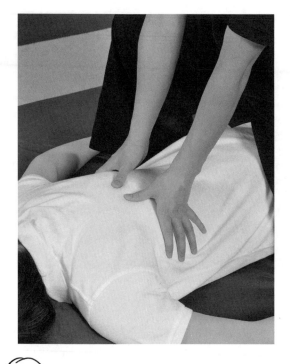

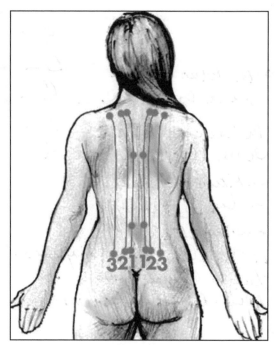

321 123

93. **Thumb Press** *Sen* **of the Back**

80/20 *presionan con los dedos
gordos, al lado de la
columna.

* Luego un poquito más lejos
como segunda linea.

* Luego más lejos
es la tercera linea

* Buscan arriba de la espalda
tocan el hueso.
usar el dedo gordo se
presionan con los 2 dedos
luego circulos cuando se
tocan las costillas.

* Luego compresiones.

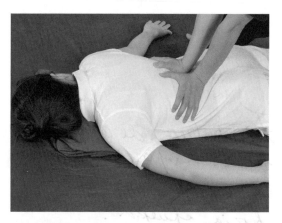

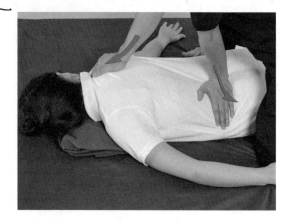

Finish the A-B-C-B-A pattern by repeating
the palm press and stretch.

Day 4

94. Palm Circle Rib Cage

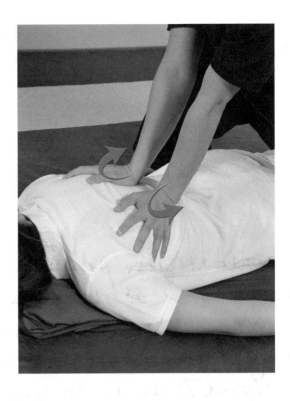

95. Pull Trapezius Muscle

Las 2 manos sobre el
Trapezius. luego jalar 2 vees.
luego pasar la mano suave.

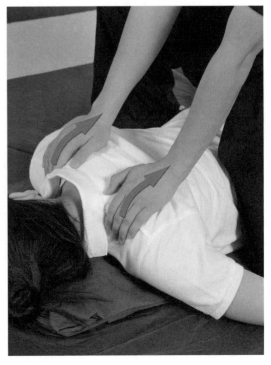

96. Shoulder Mobilization

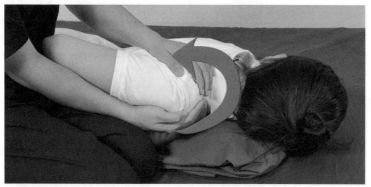

* arrodillase parelelo
* agarro el ~~E~~ brazo sobre la cintura
* Luego agarrar el hombro. con la mano derecha
* La mano izquierda sobre la escapula.
* Mover Todo el cuerpo Cuando rotamos
  a has la escapula

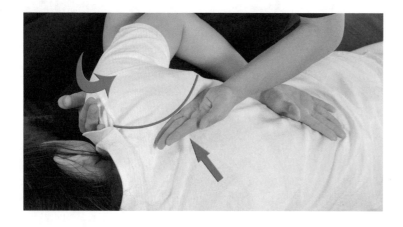

Day 4

97. Press Under Scapula

+ Siempre Comenzar sobre los pies.

* Luego el dedo gordo sobre e inside de la escapula.

* La mano derecha presiona en la mano del Cliente.

* Usar el dedo gordo. O el codo.

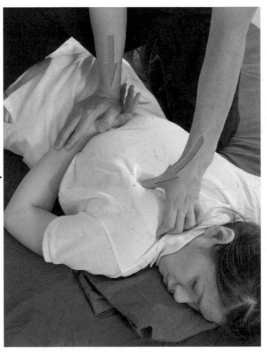

ALTERNATE METHOD

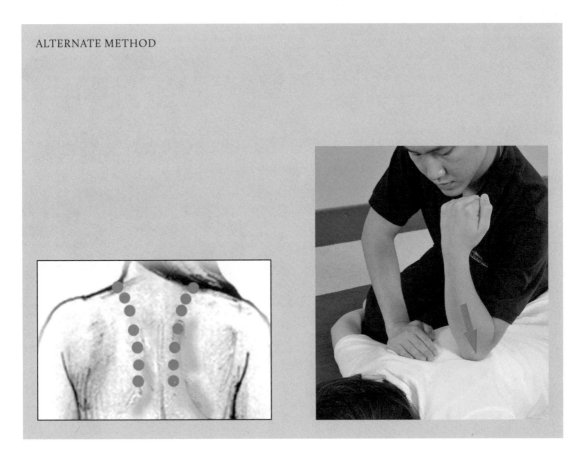

98. Cobra

* arrodíllense luego
poner las canillas Sobre
los riñones, el cuerpo
derecho.
agarren los brazos
decir el Cliente
que Mire hacia arriba
luego estirar y usar
los hombros <u>derecho</u>

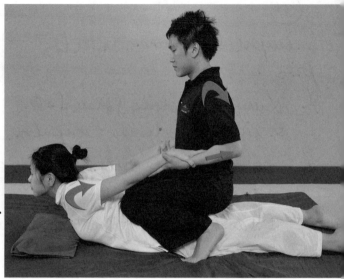

Correct alignment

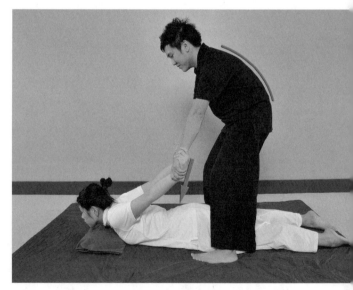

Incorrect alignment

ADVANCED VARIATION: **The King Cobra**

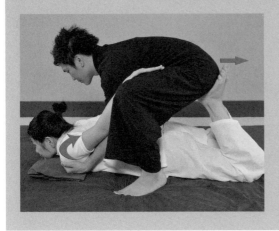 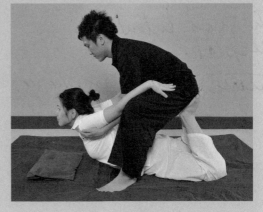

99. Single-Leg Locust

* Agarren el pie —
estirarlo suavemente
luego pisar el hueco
de los glúteos y
luego estirar la
pierna hacia arriba.

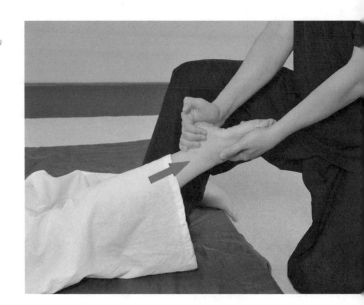

Terminar con Compresiones

* Luego lavarse las
manos antes de empezar
la cabeza.
Decirle al cliente que
voy a lavarme las manos.

* With good intentions
y respect.

* Sentarse y cruzar las piernas

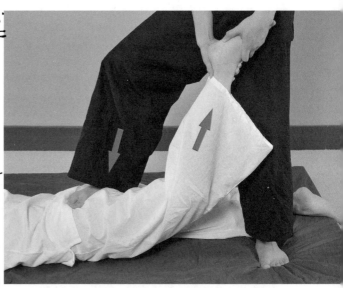

Skip

VARIATIONS: **For More Flexible Clients**

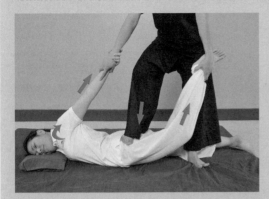 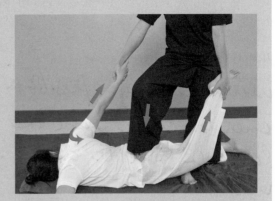

Day 4
— Head 7 Minutes —

Head, Neck, and Face Series

100. Thumb Press Under Clavicles

* *sentarse en yoga position.*
* *poner los manos sobre la clavicula Usar los dedos gordos.*

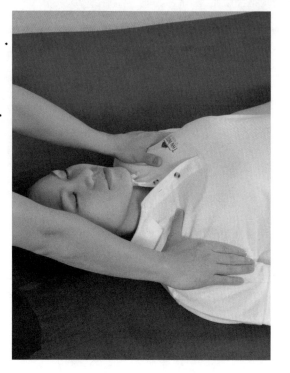

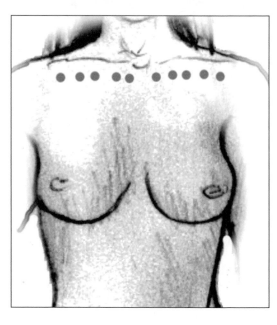

101. Gently Stretch Neck by Pressing on Shoulders

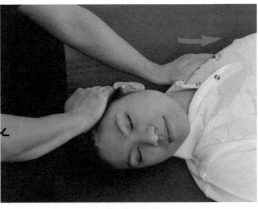

* presionar la sien suave
* presionar hacia abajo
* presionar luego en direccion de los pies.
* luego con los dedos en circulos empezando en la parte baja del cuello.
* Llegar al oido. luego masajear el oido. sepala suave.

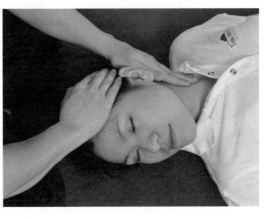

* Luego levantar la cabeza ponerla d otro lado.
* empujar dar
* empujar hacia los pies.
* Massje en circulos
* llegar al oido, luego masajear.

102. Ear Massage

Repeat Steps **101-102** for the other side.

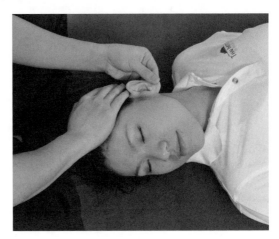

Day 4

103. Finger Press Along Trapezius and Neck

- Peuu la Cabega derecha.
Toca los Trapezius.
Masajear en circulos.
hasta llegar al occipital.
2 lineas.

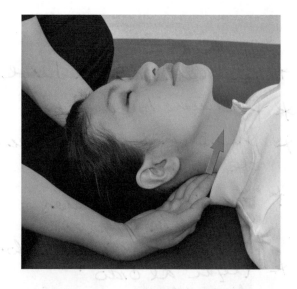

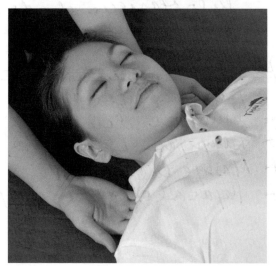

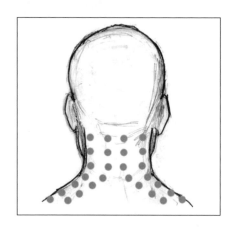

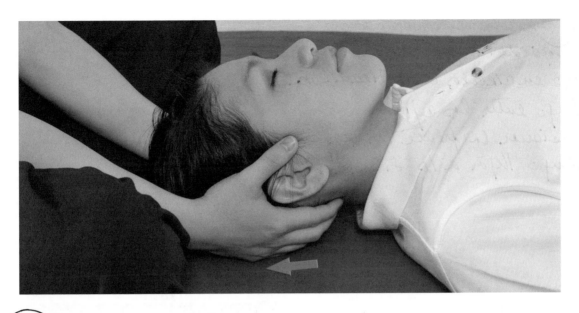

104. Base of Skull and Back of Head

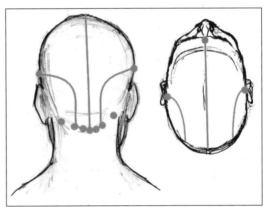

✻ Empezar en el centro de
occipital
Del centro hasta las sienes
en circulos
✻ ✝ Traccion FIRST
✻ Luego presionar de occipital.
directo hasta la frente.

Day 4

105. Forehead and Chin Lines

* dibujo de la quijada ①
* luego en circulos en la Mandibula ②
* luego entre las cejas.
* presionar la frente tres veces.
* Luego llegar a las sienes.

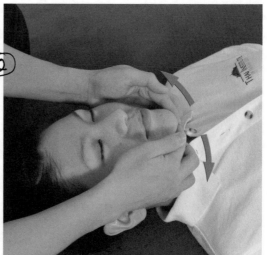

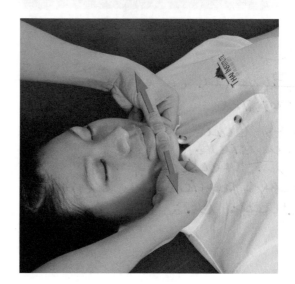

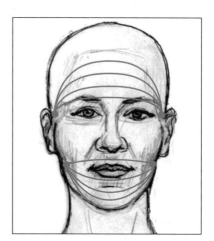

106. Scrub Scalp with "Shampooing"
     Motion

* Masajear la cabeza
de abajo hacia arriba.
* Shampooing * .

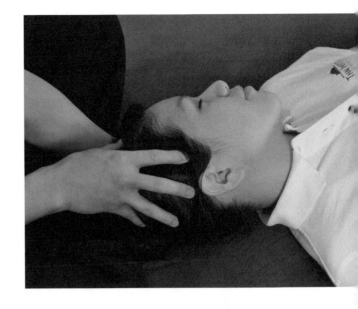

107. Create a Vacuum with the Ears

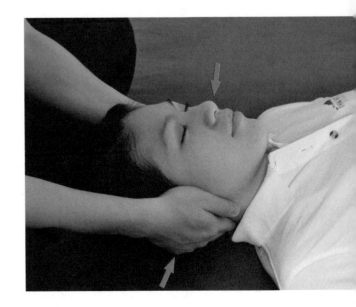

Day 4.

108. Finish with a Meditation of Thanksgiving and Healing

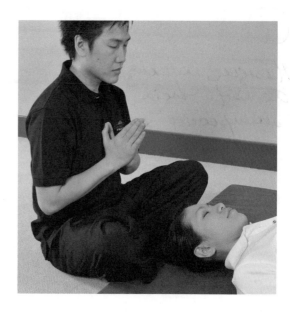

Optional steps for completing the session

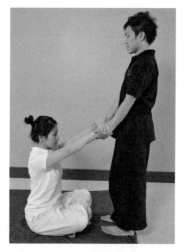

Cross-Legged Pull-Up to Seated Position

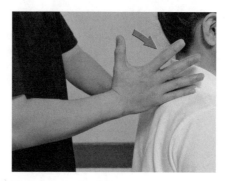

Thai Chop on Back

2.

Variations & Advanced Steps

Variations for Side Position

1. Foot Points and Leg lines

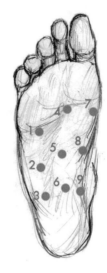 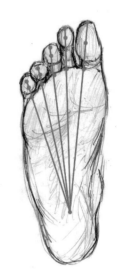

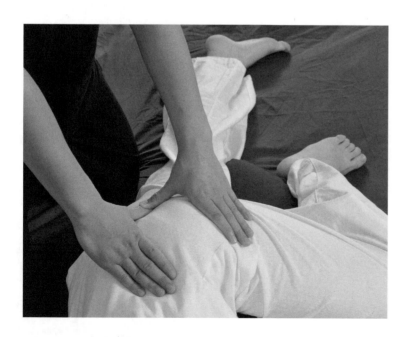 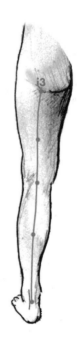

2. "Paddleboat"

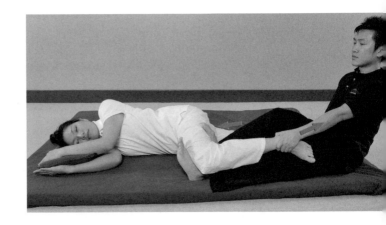

3. Finger Press

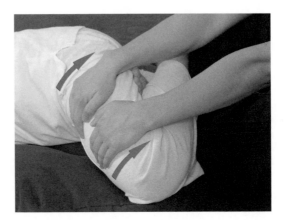

4. Hip Points

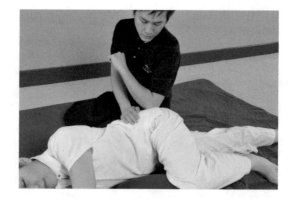

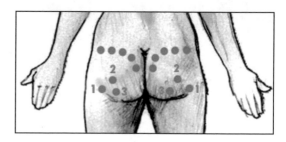

5. Back Lines

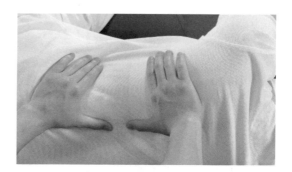

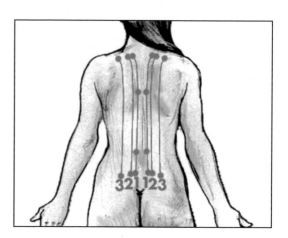

6. Shoulder Mobilization

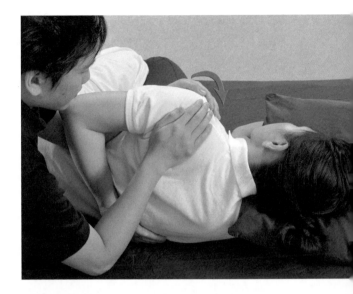

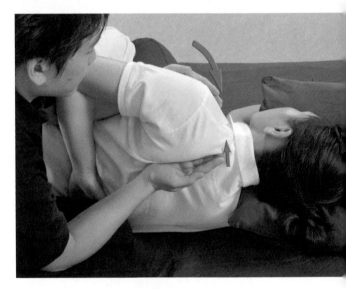

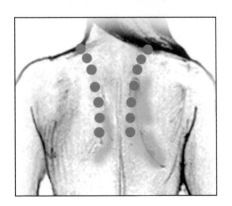

7. Triceps Stretch

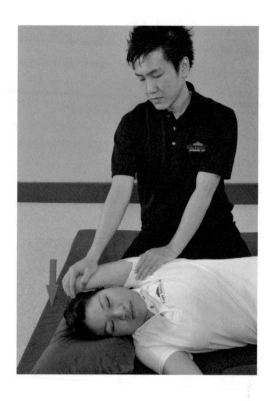

8. Rotate Shoulder and Pull Arm

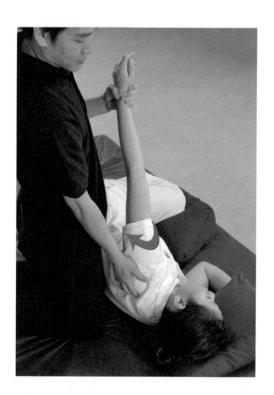

9. Arm Cross-Pull

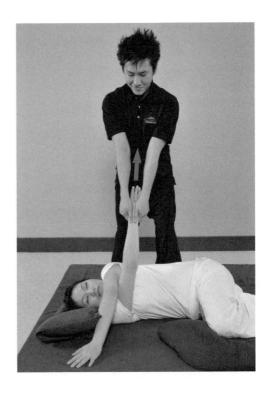

10. Basic Back Stretch

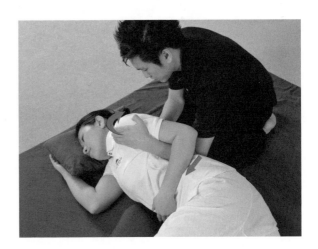

11. Locust Variations

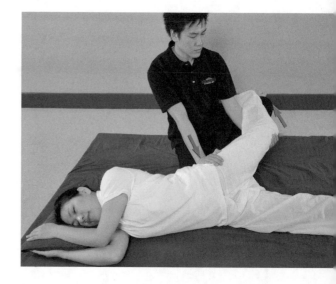

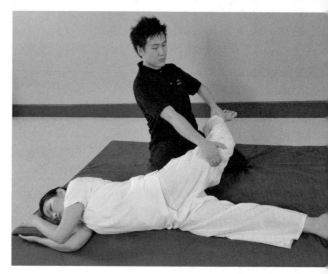

VARIATIONS:
For More Flexible Clients

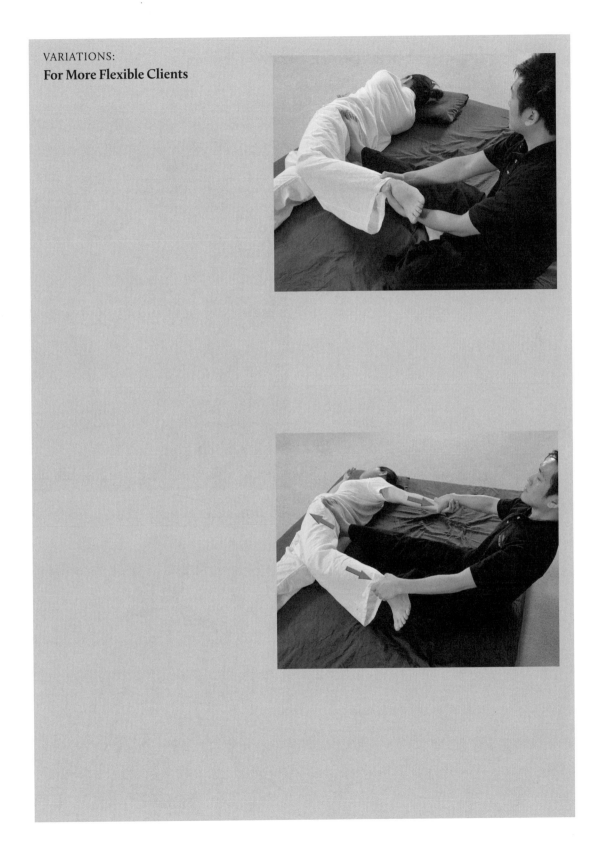

Variations for Seated Position

1. Thumb Press Back Lines

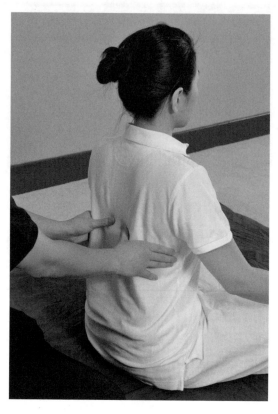

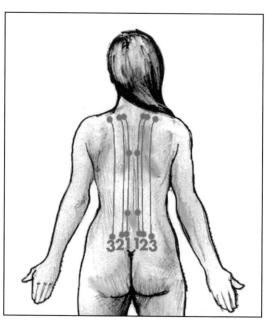

2. Scapula Mobilization

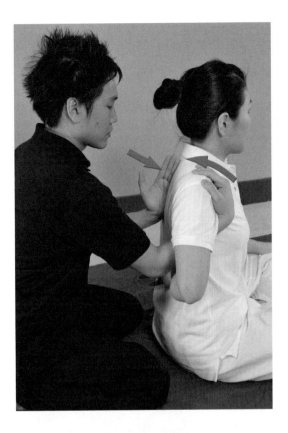

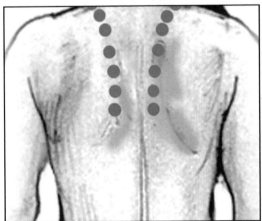

3. Triceps Routine

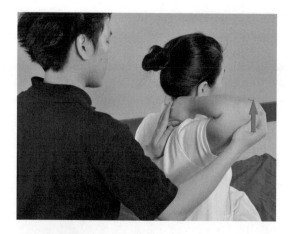

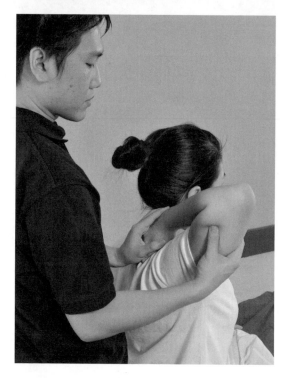

VARIATION: **For Clients Who Enjoy More Pressure**

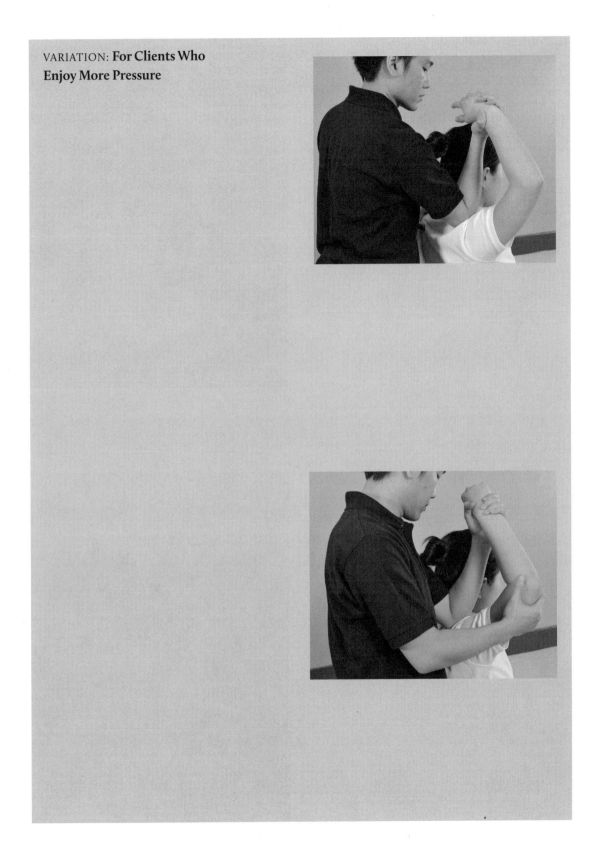

4. Rotate and Pull Arm

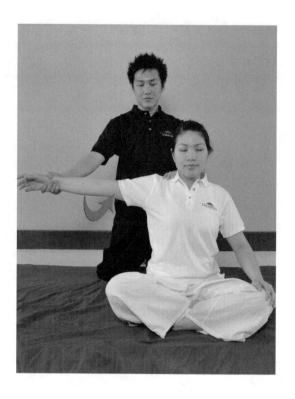

5. Thumb Press Trapezius

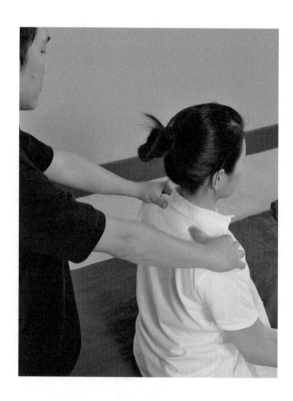

6. **Trapezius and Neck Stretch**

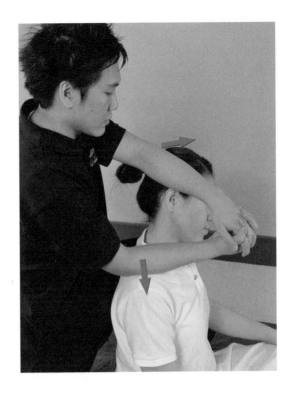

7. **Side and Neck Stretch**

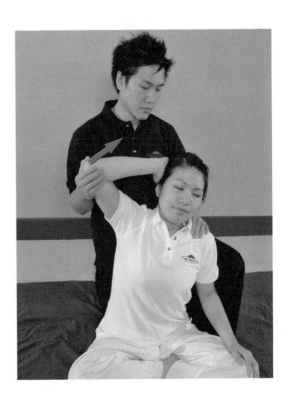

8. Thumb Press Neck Points

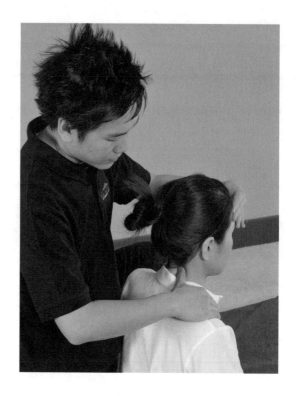

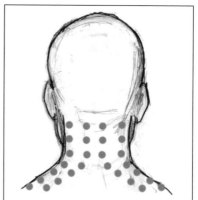

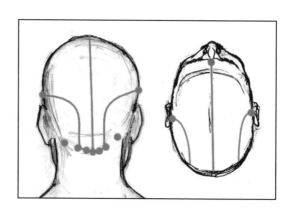

9. Face Massage

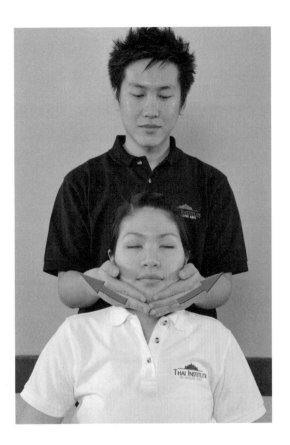

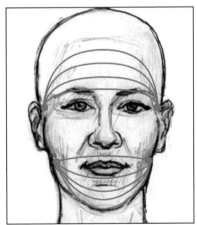

Advanced Postures

1. Advanced Back Stretch

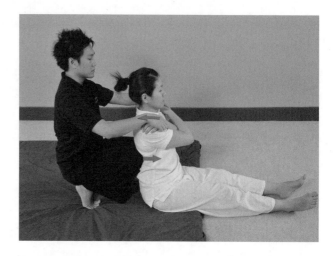

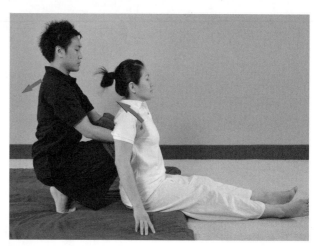

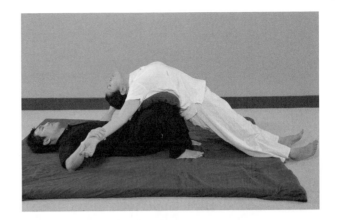

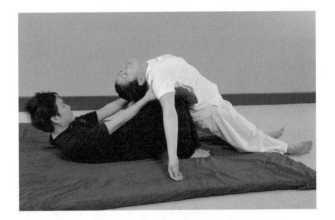

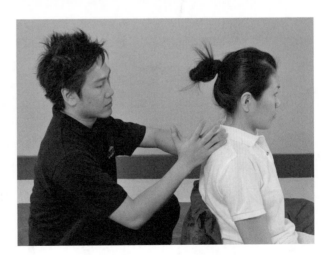

2. Bridge Pose

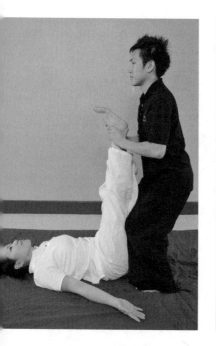 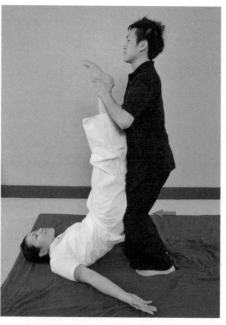 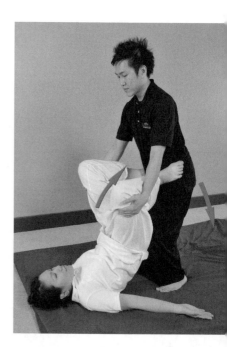

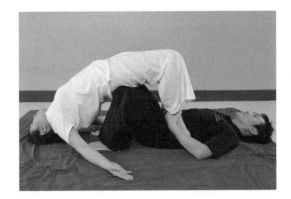

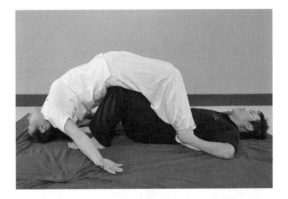

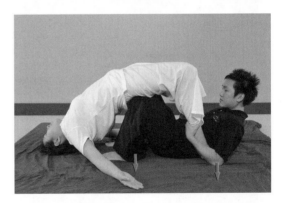

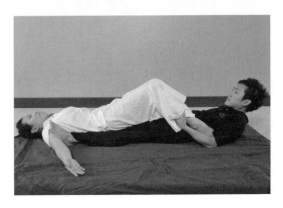

3. Shoulder Stand

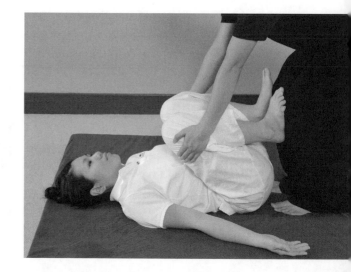

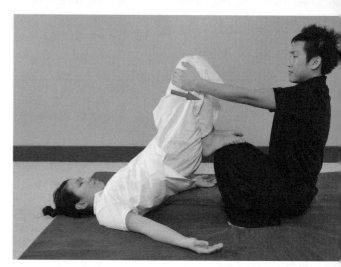

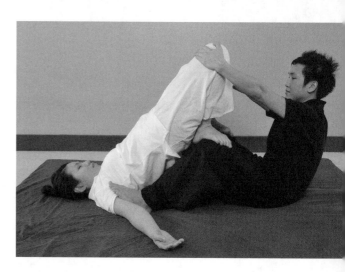

4. Full Locust

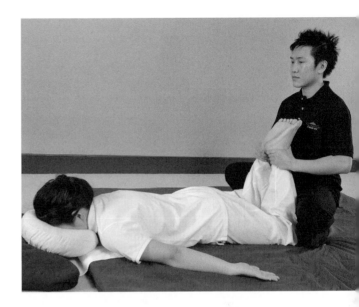

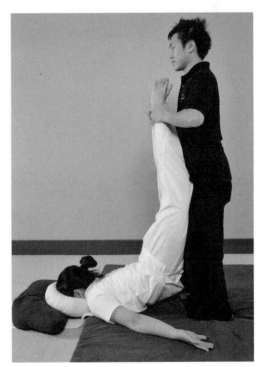

Walking Massage

1. Walking Frog

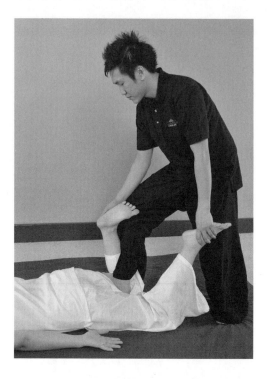

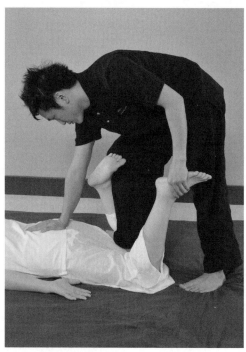

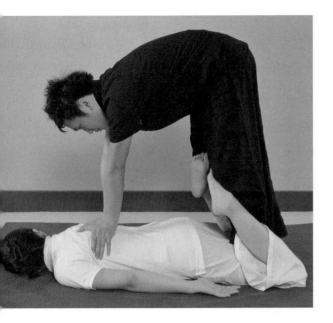

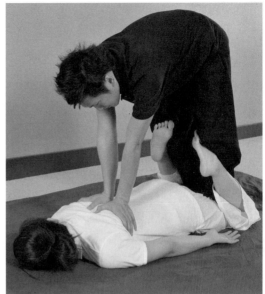

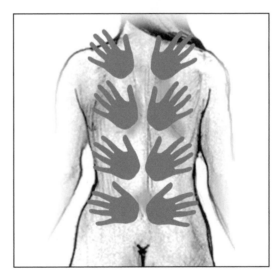

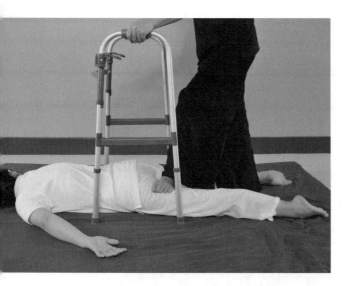

2. Walking on the Back with One Foot

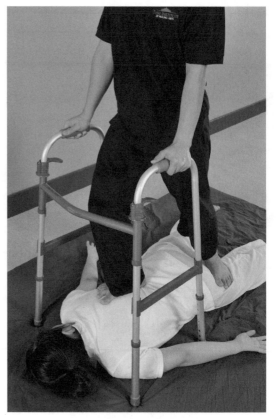

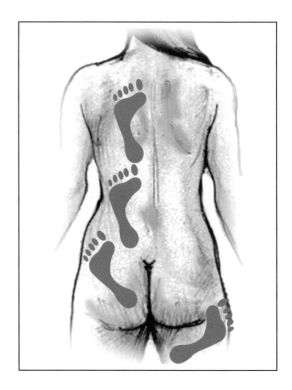

3. Walking on the Back with Two Feet

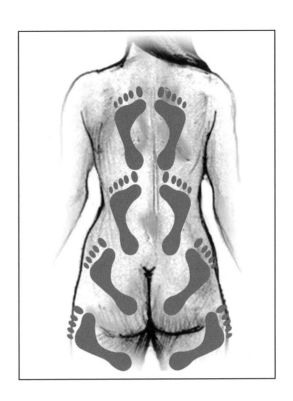

3.

Resources

An Introduction to Traditional Thai Medicine

EXCERPT FROM *THAI HERBAL MEDICINE (SECOND EDITION).*

Traditional Thai Medicine advocates the holistic combination of three approaches: therapies for the body, mind-heart, and energy. According this philosophy, body therapies are approaches that affect the concrete substances that make up our physical self, traditionally thought of in terms of the Four Elements Earth, Water, Fire, and Air. Mind-heart (the Thai term is *citta*) means both the intellect and the emotions. This word refers to the entire gamut of thoughts, emotions, and intuitions that make us the individuals we are. The mind-heart is separate from but intimately tied to the physical body, and in the Thai system it is energy (*lom* in Thai) that holds these together. Roughly analogous to the Chinese idea of *qi* (or *chi*) and to the Indian concept of *prana*, this energy is an intangible flow that moves through the body via specific channels or pathways called *sen*. The Thai model recognizes 72,000 of these *sen*, which run throughout the body connecting certain anatomical landmarks. The Thai healing arts can be split into three distinct approaches that each encompass one of the above approaches...

Body Therapy: Dietary regimens and herbal medicine

Herbs and food affect the human organism by causing physiological changes in body chemistry, and therefore these are considered to be primarily therapies for the physical body. This does not mean that the effects of these therapies are limited only to the physical body. Because of the intimate link between body, mind and energy, a traditional Thai doctor can encourage healing processes within the physical, mental and energetic selves by prescribing therapeutic herbs, minerals, and other natural substances. However, solutions to physical problems are usually sought in dietary changes first, and old Thai axiom states that "the cause of disease is in the stomach." Thai herbalists typically use concentrated herbal medicines only as a last resort. When such medicines are prescribed, they are always administered in conjunction with dietary recommendations. By understanding the properties of foods, the traditional Thai doctor teaches patients to harmonize their diets with their constitutions and the environment in order to avoid future imbalance that lead to illness. For more information on Thai herbal medicine, please see *Thai Herbal Medicine*, available from Findhorn Press.

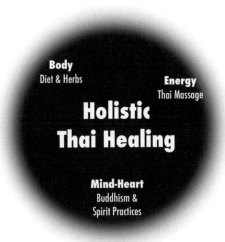

Mind-Heart Therapy: Spiritual healing

Spiritual healing (including both religious and magical therapies) remains prevalent in Thailand today, even in the most modernized cities. Thai medicine emphasizes the spiritual well-being of the patient, and holds that many diseases flow from a troubled mind-heart. For this reason, Thai medicine incorporates a diverse selection of both Buddhist and shamanic practices designed to heal emotional and psychological disorders. In Thailand, spiritual healing often involves elaborate rituals that emphasize the importance of the patient's relationships with family, friends, and the community in the healing process. Meditations, chanting, breathing techniques, and visualizations drawn from Buddhist tradition are used for relaxation and treatment of anxiety. In addition, magic spells, healing amulets, and the exorcism of evil spirits drawn from both Buddhism and indigenous Thai culture also play a major role in contemporary Thai spiritual healing. For more information on Thai spiritual healing, please see *Traditional Thai Medicine: Buddhism, Animism, Ayurveda*, available from Hohm Press.

Energy Therapy: Thai Massage

Thai massage is not considered to be bodywork, but rather is seen in Thailand primarily a therapy of energy. Therapists do not soothe muscles with stroking Swedish-like movements, but rather apply acupressure to certain points on the body in order to increase the flow of energy through the *sen* as necessary to relieve symptoms and stimulate healing. These techniques can only be understood by studying where the *sen* run within the body, and which systems they affect. While Thai massage has enjoyed increasing popularity in the West as of late, it is a field that, in Thailand, remains intimately tied to the other three branches of traditional medicine. Part of the purpose of this series of books by Dr. C. Pierce Salguero is to introduce traditional Thai medicine as a whole, as a framework through which Thai massage can be seen in a more holistic context. For more information on Thai massage therapy, please see *Encyclopedia of Thai Massage (Second Edition)*, available from Findhorn Press.

Sen Lines & Acupressure Points for Thai Massage

EXCERPT FROM *ENCYCLOPEDIA OF THAI MASSAGE (SECOND EDITION)*.

Sen

The concept of invisible energy meridians coursing throughout the body is common to most Asian medical traditions. Of these traditions, the energy meridians most well known in the West are those used in Traditional Chinese Medicine (TCM). The Thai energy meridians, or *sen* as they are called in Thai, do have some similarities with Chinese and Indian lines. However, while they have been influenced by these ideas, the *sen* are uniquely Thai. Thai Massage therapists must learn the *sen* in order to perform the techniques properly and not rely on knowledge of other traditions.

It is said in the Thai tradition that there are **72,000** *sen*. This number should not be taken literally, however, as it is a way of saying "an infinite amount." The point is that every part of the body is linked to every other part through an infinite and intricate mesh of energy. This energy is known as *prana* (Sanskrit), *qi* or *chi* (Chinese), or *lom* (Thai). In Thai thinking, the *sen* make up an energy network that permeates the body of all living beings, and that vibrates in response to physiological, psychological, and spiritual experiences. According to the traditional understanding, this energy also emanates beyond the body, creating a field around the organism commonly referred to as an aura.

No one can name and diagram all of the body's infinite energy circuits. However, **10** main *sen* are commonly taught and used in treatment by the Shivagakomarpaj Lineage. These **10** *sen* are the main conduits, or "high-ways," of energy in the body, from which the rest of the *sen* branch. As a result, when they are treated, benefits emanate through the entire system. While many *sen* systems exist in Thailand, this book is based on the model taught by the Shivagakomarpaj Lineage of Thai massage.

Acupressure Techniques

Acupressure points are shown on the diagrams on the next pages to indicate spots which are particularly powerful for stimulating energy flow. When treating specific diseases and disorders, the entire correlating *sen* should be treated, and all acupressure points should be activated. You will note that some of the diagrams include smaller lines branching off of the main *sen*. These important branches are always massaged in conjunction with the main energy lines, and should not be forgotten. The following three steps should be followed for application of acupressure to each point on the body:

1. Before acupressure is applied to a point, the point should be warmed up with five clockwise and five counterclockwise thumb circles.
2. Acupressure should be given with thumb presses. Pressure should be applied with the pad of the thumb, perpendicularly to the surface of the skin. (See Chapter **3** for proper body mechanics for thumb press.) Each point should be pressed three times. Each time, the therapist should begin with slowly increasing pressure over a period of **5** seconds. Maximum pressure should be held for **2** or **3** seconds. The pressure should be lifted slowly over **2** or **3** seconds, for a total of about **10** seconds per point.
3. After acupressure, the point should be soothed with five clockwise and five counterclockwise thumb circles.

Never use acupressure on other parts of the body, bone surfaces, recent injuries, or other sensitive areas of the body.

Hot & Cold Pressure

Two major problems can occur with the *sen*: breakage and blockage. The difference between the breakage and blockage of a *sen* is often difficult to discern for a beginning practitioner. In both cases, the client will typically report pain as the major symptom. It is important to differentiate between the two, however, since this will determine how you administer your therapy.

Sen Breaks

The main causes of a *sen* break are muscle strains, tendon sprains, nerve pain, bruises, and bone injuries. *Sen* breaks are almost always acute conditions, brought on by a sudden injury, and need immediate attention. Traditionally it is said that broken *sen* cause energy to escape the channel and pool in the surrounding tissue, typically producing sharp, shooting pain. Breaks thus will be accompanied by swelling, redness, and sensitivity in the area around the injury.

Sen breaks are said to require "cold treatment." The word "cold" is being used here both literally and metaphorically. Ice packs or cold herbal compresses should be applied to the body part, and the massage practitioner should apply only indirect or "cold" pressure to this area.

Cold pressure is a technique to help dissipate pooled energy away from the affected area in order to allow the break to heal. Light thumb presses should be applied to the *sen* above and below the break, and should move outward from the affected area all the way to the ends of the *sen* or segment. The practitioner should take care to never press toward or directly on the broken *sen*, as this will cause an increase in pooled energy rather than contribute to its dissipation. Should the client experience pain at any time, use a lighter touch.

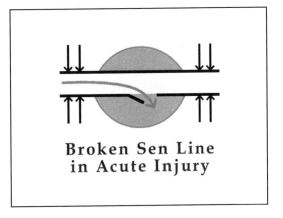

Broken Sen Line in Acute Injury

The diagram above shows a broken *sen* with localized swelling in red. Black arrows indicate where pressure should be applied. Never apply pressure directly to the swollen area.

After **48** hours, a *sen* breakage will have begun to mend, and the swelling and heat will typically have subsided. At this point, cold therapy should be replaced by hot therapy. The injury should be treated as a blockage in order to clear out stagnated energy and get things flowing properly again.

Sen Blockages

Blocked *sen* are usually chronic conditions caused by fatigue, stress, bad posture, repetitive stress, or previous injuries. Blockages usually manifest as muscle knots, tendonitis, localized stiffness, and soreness, but they can also be characterized by dull pain, weakness, stiffness, numbness, and sometimes even paralysis. Blockages are explained as obstructions in the *sen* that cause the flow of energy to organs and limbs farther along the channel to be inhibited. They are metaphorically analogous to cholesterol buildup in the arteries.

Sen blockages are treated with hot therapy, which includes application of hot compresses, hot baths or saunas with spicy and aromatic herbs, and "hot pressure." Hot pressure is acupressure applied directly to the location of the blockage with strong intensity in order to break up the obstruction and increase free flow of energy.

Typically, hot acupressure is given with thumb presses, but some clients may require (or prefer) the use of the elbow, knee, or heel press on the site of a blockage. Always remember that care must be taken not to injure the client with these more intensive techniques. *Sen* are particularly vulnerable at a site of blockage, and too much pressure may in fact cause a breakage. If a client is experiencing too much pain to effectively apply pressure to the blockage, hot compresses may be used instead.

Whatever method you use, apply pressure to the site of the blockage, and then to move along the *sen* away from the site, as if "flushing" the blockage away. Travel all the way to the ends of the *sen* or *sen* segment, and return by pressing toward the site. Travel through the site and continue to the opposite end of the segment. Then return back to the site once again. This encourages the disposal of stagnated energy and the flow of fresh energy in both directions. Blockages also respond well to Opening the Wind Gates.

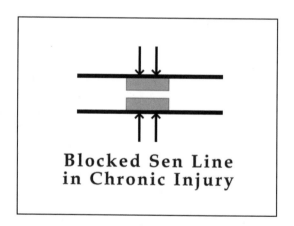

Blocked Sen Line in Chronic Injury

The diagram above shows a blocked *sen*. Arrows indicate where pressure should be applied, directly on the blockage.

The charts on the following pages are excerpted from the *Encyclopedia of Thai Massage (Second Edition)* from Findhorn Press. For more information on therapies, contraindication, and more, please consult that book.

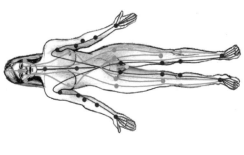
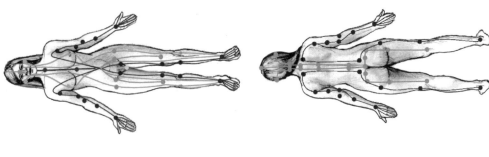

ABDOMINAL PAIN/DISEASE/DISORDERS (LOWER): Itha-Pingala, Kalatharee, Sahatsarangsi-Tawaree

ABDOMINAL PAIN/DISEASE/DISORDERS (UPPER): Sumana

ACID REFLUX: Sumana

ANGINA: Kalatharee

ANXIETY: Itha-Pingala

APPENDICITIS: Sahatsarangsi-Tawaree

ARM PAIN/STIFFNESS/INJURY: Kalatharee

ARTHRITIS (OF LIMBS, DIGITS): Kalatharee

ASTHMA: Sumana

BACK PAIN/STIFFNESS/INJURY: Itha-Pingala

BELL'S PALSY: Sahatsarangsi-Tawaree, Lawusang-Ulanga

BIPOLAR DISORDER: Sahatsarangsi-Tawaree

BLOOD PRESSURE: Itha-Pingala

BREAST DISEASE/DISORDER/CANCER: Lawusang-Ulanga

BREATHING, DIFFICULTY OF: Sumana

BRONCHITIS: Sumana

CARDIAC ARRHYTHMIA: Kalatharee

CARDIAC DISEASE/DISORDER: Kalatharee

CATARACTS: Sahatsarangsi-Tawaree

CHEST PAIN: Kalatharee, Sahatsarangsi-Tawaree, Sumana, Lawusang-Ulanga

CHILL: Itha-Pingala

COLD: Itha-Pingala, Sumana

COLON PAIN/DISEASE/DISORDERS: Itha-Pingala, Kalatharee, Sahatsarangsi-Tawaree, Nantakawat

CONSTIPATION: Nantakawat

COUGH: Itha-Pingala, Kalatharee, Sumana

CRAMPS, MENSTRUAL: Nantakawat

CRAMPS, OF ABDOMEN: Sahatsarangsi-Tawaree

CRAMPS, OF LEG: Sahatsarangsi-Tawaree

DEPRESSION: Kalatharee

DIAPHRAGM SPASM/DISORDER: Sumana

DIARRHEA: Nantakawat

DIZZINESS: Itha-Pingala

EAR INFECTION/DISEASE/DISORDER: Lawusang-Ulanga

EPILEPSY: Kalatharee

ERECTILE DYSFUNCTION: Kitcha

EYE, INFECTION OF: Sahatsarangsi-Tawaree

EYES: Itha-Pingala, Sahatsarangsi-Tawaree

FACIAL PARALYSIS: Sahatsarangsi-Tawaree, Lawusang-Ulanga

FATIGUE: Itha-Pingala, Sahatsarangsi-Tawaree

FEVER: Itha-Pingala, Sahatsarangsi-Tawaree

FINGER PAIN/STIFFNESS/INJURY: Kalatharee

FOOT PAIN/STIFFNESS/INJURY: Kalatharee

GALL BLADDER DISEASE/DISORDERS: Itha-Pingala

GASTROINTESTINAL PAIN/DISEASE/DISORDERS (LOWER): Itha-Pingala, Kalatharee, Sahatsarangsi-Tawaree, Nantakawat

GASTROINTESTINAL PAIN/DISEASE/DISORDERS (UPPER): Sumana, Lawusang-Ulanga

GLAUCOMA: Sahatsarangsi-Tawaree

GUM DISEASE: Sahatsarangsi-Tawaree

HAND PAIN/STIFFNESS/INJURY: Kalatharee

HEADACHE: Itha-Pingala

HEARING LOSS: Lawusang-Ulanga

HEART DISEASE: Kalatharee, Sumana

HERNIA: Kalatharee, Sahatsarangsi-Tawaree, Kitcha

INCONTINENCE: Nantakawat

INDIGESTION: Sumana

INFERTILITY: Kitcha

INSOMNIA: Sahatsarangsi-Tawaree

INTESTINAL DISEASE/DISORDERS: Itha-Pingala, Kalatharee, Sahatsarangsi-Tawaree, Nantakawat

JAUNDICE: Kalatharee

JAW PAIN/STIFFNESS: Lawusang-Ulanga

KNEE PAIN/STIFFNESS/INJURY: Itha-Pingala, Kalatharee, Sahatsarangsi-Tawaree

LACTATION: Lawusang-Ulanga

LEG PAIN/STIFFNESS/INJURY: Kalatharee

LETHARGY: Itha-Pingala, Sahatsarangsi-Tawaree

LIVER DISEASE/DISORDERS: Pingala

LUNGS DISEASE/DISORDER/INFECTION: Sumana, Lawusang-Ulanga

MENSTRUATION, IRREGULARITIES OR PAIN: Nantakawat

NASAL CONGESTION: Itha-Pingala

NAUSEA: Sumana

NECK PAIN/STIFFNESS/INJURY: Itha-Pingala

ORAL INFECTION: Sahatsarangsi-Tawaree

OVARIAN DISEASE/DISORDER: Kitcha

PARALYSIS (OF LIMB/S): Kalatharee

PARALYSIS (SPINAL CORD INJURY): Itha-Pingala

PEPTIC ULCER: Sumana

PROSTATE DISEASE/DISORDER/CANCER: Kitcha

PSYCHOLOGICAL DISORDERS: Kalatharee

REPRODUCTIVE SYSTEM DISEASE/DISORDER: Kitcha

RESPIRATORY SYSTEM INFECTION/DISEASE/DISORDER: Sumana

RHEUMATIC HEART DISEASE: Kalatharee

SCHIZOPHRENIA: Kalatharee

SEPTUM: Itha-Pingala

SEX DRIVE, LACK OF: Kitcha

SEXUAL DYSFUNCTION: Kitcha

SHOCK: Kalatharee

SHOULDER PAIN/STIFFNESS: Itha-Pingala

SINUSITIS: Itha-Pingala

SORE THROAT: Itha-Pingala, Sahatsarangsi-Tawaree, Sumana, Lawusang-Ulanga

STOMACH PAIN/DISEASE/DISORDER: Sumana, Lawusang-Ulanga

STRESS: Itha-Pingala

TESTICULAR DISEASE/DISORDER: Kitcha

THROAT INFECTION/DISEASE/DISORDER: Itha-Pingala, Sahatsarangsi-Tawaree, Sumana, Lawusang-Ulanga

TINNITIS: Lawusang-Ulanga

TMJ: Lawusang-Ulanga

TOE PAIN/STIFFNESS/INJURY: Kalatharee

TOOTHACHE: Sahatsarangsi-Tawaree, Lawusang-Ulanga

ULCER, PEPTIC: Sumana

URINARY TRACT INFECTION: Itha-Pingala, Nantakawat

UROGENITAL INFECTION/DISEASE/DISORDER: Itha-Pingala, Sahatsarangsi-Tawaree

UTERUS DISEASE/DISORDER: Nantakawat, Kitcha

VAGINAL INFECTION/DISEASE/DISORDER: Kitcha

VERTIGO: Itha-Pingala

VISION, IMPAIRMENT OF: Itha-Pingala, Sahatsarangsi-Tawaree

VOMITING: Sumana

WEAKNESS: Itha-Pingala, Sahatsarangsi-Tawaree

WHOOPING COUGH: Kalatharee

Sen Lines, Acupressure Points, and Correlations for Thai Massage Therapy

Thai Acupressure for Hands & Feet

HAND AND FOOT MASSAGE: The acupressure points in the hands and feet stimulate energy flow throughout the body. These acupressure points are used in treatment of any disorders or diseases.

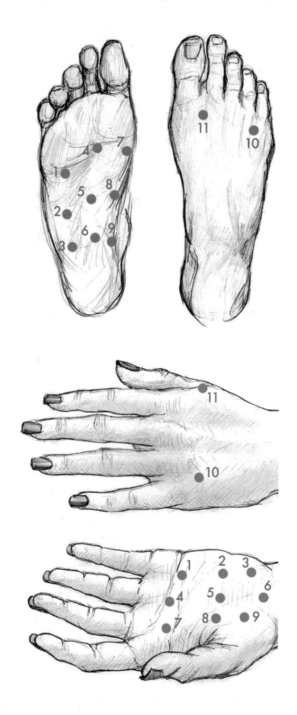

Sen Segments in Arms & Legs

ARM AND LEG MASSAGE: In the classic routine, rather than following specific *sen* lines throughout the body, all sen lines in a particular body part are massaged before moving on to another area. Thumb press the sen segments passing through the arms and legs.

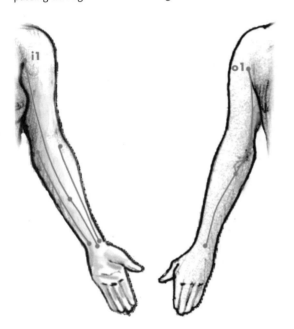

Sen **Segments in Arms:** The outer arm line (**o1**) runs along the posterior side of the arm, beginning at the center of the wrist joint. It runs in between the radius and the ulna, along the medial side of the humerus, and ends at the center of the back of the shoulder on the outer edge of the scapula. The inner arm line (**i1**) runs along the anterior side of the arm from the wrist joint, up the middle of the forearm, through the elbow, along the medial side of the humerus, and ends at the center of the armpit. Two branches of this line begin at the wrist and run along the medial side of the radius and ulna respectively, widening slightly before terminating at the crease in the elbow.

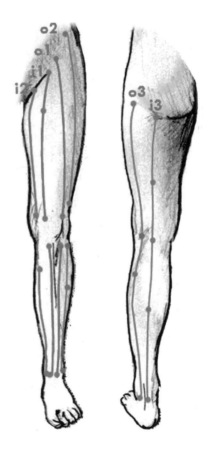

Sen **Segments in Legs:** On the medial side of the leg, the first inner leg line (**i1**) runs from the ankle, along the medial side of the tibia, through the medial side of the knee, along the medial side of the femur, and ends at the top of the quadriceps. The second inner leg line (**i2**) runs from between the medial side of the ankle and the Achilles tendon, along the medial side of the calf and thigh, and ends at the groin. The third inner leg line (**i3**) runs along the posterior side of the leg from the top of the Achilles tendon, up the midline of the calf and hamstring, to end at the top of the femur.

On the lateral side of the leg, the first outer leg line (**o1**) runs from the front of the ankle, along the lateral side of the intercondylar eminence of the tibia, through the lateral side of the knee, along the lateral side of the femur, to end at the hip flexor. The second outer leg line (**o2**) runs from the outside of the ankle, up the lateral side of the calf, along the tensor fasciae latae, to end at the head of the femur. The third outer leg line (**o3**) begins between the ankle and Achilles tendon, travels up the outside edge of the calf, along the lateral edge of the hamstring, to end at the gluteal crease.

Sen Segments in Back & Hips

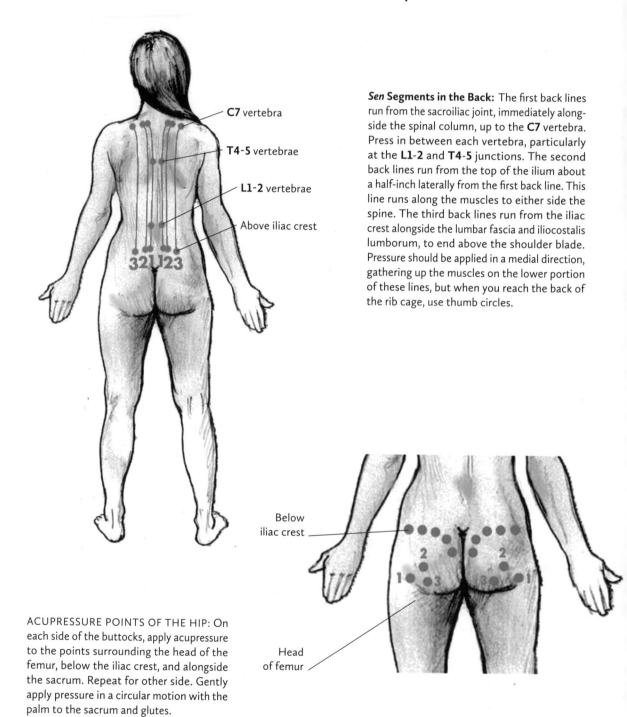

C7 vertebra

T4-5 vertebrae

L1-2 vertebrae

Above iliac crest

321|23

Sen Segments in the Back: The first back lines run from the sacroiliac joint, immediately alongside the spinal column, up to the **C7** vertebra. Press in between each vertebra, particularly at the **L1-2** and **T4-5** junctions. The second back lines run from the top of the ilium about a half-inch laterally from the first back line. This line runs along the muscles to either side the spine. The third back lines run from the iliac crest alongside the lumbar fascia and iliocostalis lumborum, to end above the shoulder blade. Pressure should be applied in a medial direction, gathering up the muscles on the lower portion of these lines, but when you reach the back of the rib cage, use thumb circles.

Below iliac crest

2   2

1   3   3   1

Head of femur

ACUPRESSURE POINTS OF THE HIP: On each side of the buttocks, apply acupressure to the points surrounding the head of the femur, below the iliac crest, and alongside the sacrum. Repeat for other side. Gently apply pressure in a circular motion with the palm to the sacrum and glutes.

Sen Itha & Pingala

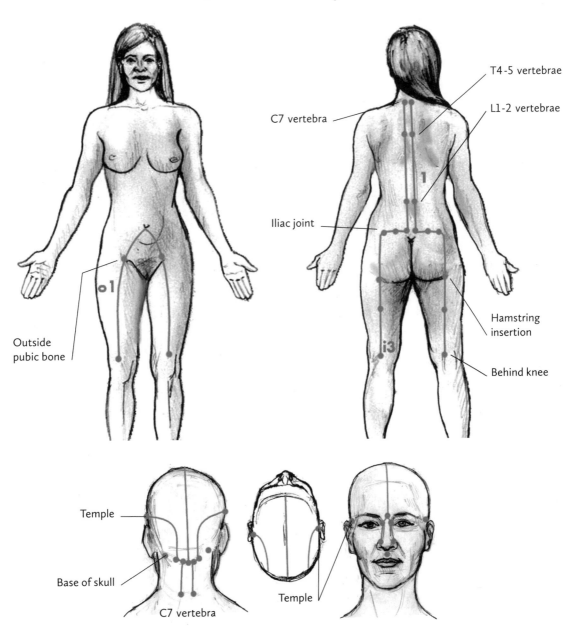

Itha and Pingala: The Itha (left side) and Pingala (right side) begin at the navel, run down the first outer leg line (**o1**), turn at the knee, run up the third inner leg line (**i3**), along the top of the iliac crest, and up along the first back line (**1**). The portion of **o1** and **i3** below the knee are considered secondary branch lines, but should be worked as part of this sen.

At the base of the skull, the two sen become three, with outer branches terminating at the temples, and the inner branch continuing over the top of the head, branching again at the third eye, and terminating at the nostrils.

The Itha and Pingala sen are used to treat the back, knees, head, nose, and sinuses.

Sen Kalatharee

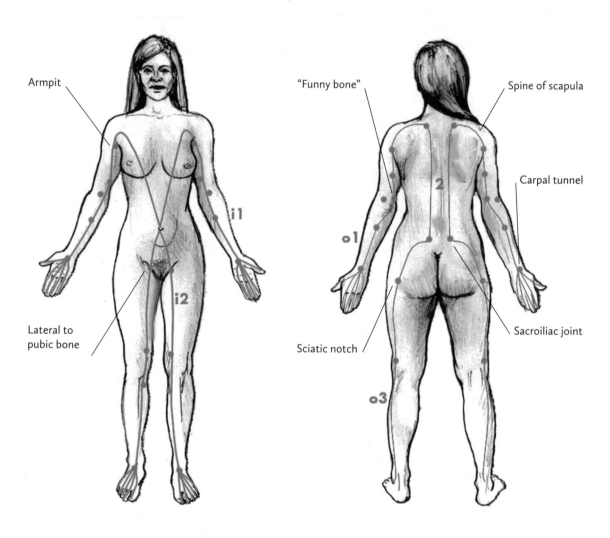

Armpit

"Funny bone"

Spine of scapula

Carpal tunnel

i1

i2

Lateral to
pubic bone

Sacroiliac joint

Sciatic notch

o1

2

o3

Kalatharee: The Kalatharee runs from the navel in four branches. It descends along the second inner leg lines (**i2**) and ascends along the inner arm lines (**i1**), terminating at the toes and fingers. Kalatharee is reflected on the back side of the limbs along the third outer leg lines (**o3**) and the outer arm lines (**o1**). The Kalatharee is shown in most diagrams with a section of this sen running through the back along the second back line (**2**), running slightly lateral to Itha and Pingala. Kalatharee is used to treat the heart, chest, and limbs, as well as psychological and spiritual balance.

Sen Sahatsarangsi & Tawaree

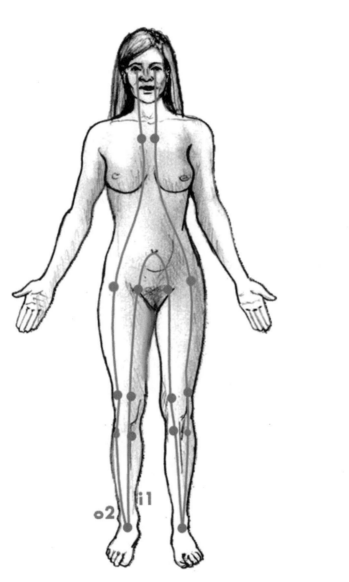

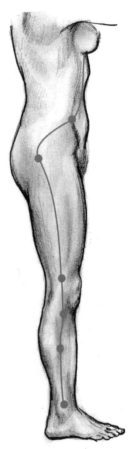

Sahatsarangsi and Tawaree: The Sahatsarangsi (left side) and Tawaree (right side) run from the navel, descend the first inner leg line (**i1**), turn at the ankle, ascend the second outer leg line (**o2**), through the pelvic girdle, up the chest, and terminate at the eyes. These sen are used to treat the eyes, the lower abdominal region, and the chest.

Sen Sumana, Lawusang & Ulanga

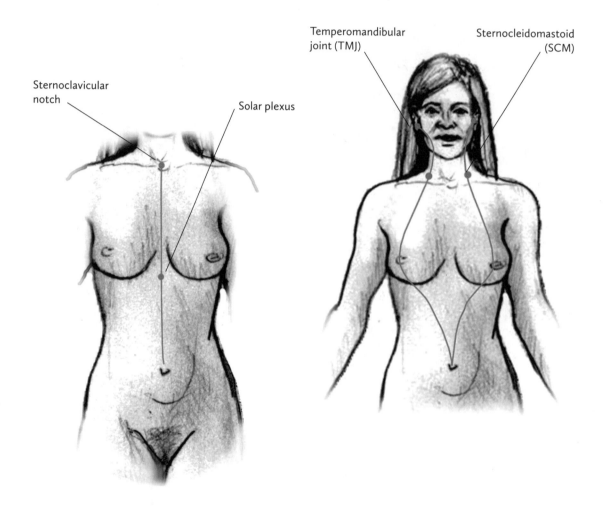

Sumana: The Sumana runs from the navel to the base of the tongue. The Sumana is used to treat the upper digestive tract, heart, lungs, and upper respiratory system. This *sen* approximately correlates to the Sushumna nadi from the yoga tradition, the sen that runs up along the inside of the spinal cord and along which are found the six chakras, or main spiritual energy centers in the body. Thus, the Sumana is seen as a very important line of energy, and can be used in the treatment of any disorder.

Lawusang and Ulanga: The Lawusang (left side) and Ulanga (right side) run from the navel through the nipple, up the side of neck, and terminate just below the ears. These sen are used to treat the breasts, ears, throat, mouth, teeth, and jaw.

Sen Nantakawat & Kitcha

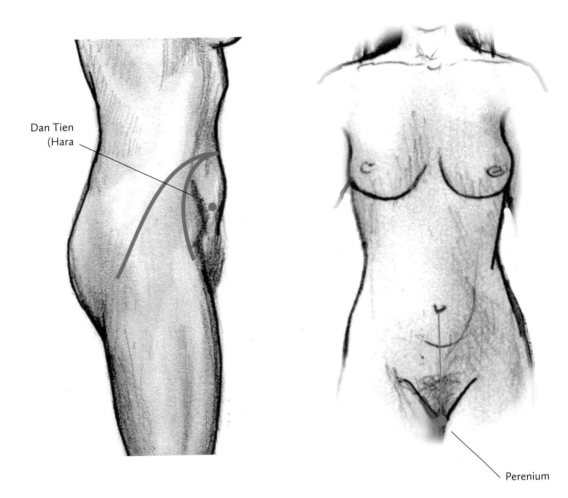

Nantakawat: The Nantakawat runs from the navel to the excretion organs in two branches. The Sikhinee runs to the urethra, and the Sukumand runs to the anus. The major acupressure point is the hara or dantian, shown in the diagram.

Kitcha: The Kitcha runs from the navel to the perineum, passing through the reproductive organs. In the male, the Kitcha is called the Pittakun, and in the female, it is called the Kitchana. It correlates to sexual function and fertility, including the testes and prostate in men and the uterus and ovaries in women. The perineum is the main acupressure point on this sen, but this point should not be treated with direct acupressure. It can be stimulated, with the patient's consent, by applying warm herbal compress.

Shivagakomarpaj Lineage

Shivagakomarpaj Lineage

The two schools mentioned below function as "sister schools," offering students the opportunity to study in the US or in Thailand while staying within the same curriculum, organizational structure, and educational philosophy. Once you complete a course at either school, you are able to repeat the same course as often as you like at either location at no additional cost. By allowing students to be present in the classroom continuously without additional cost, this free internship program allows students the opportunity to approximate the experience of an immersion-style learning over the long term. (See the following website to link to both locations: www.oldmedicinehospital.com.)

Thai Massage School Shivagakomarpaj ("Old Medicine Hospital") www.thaimassageschool.ac.th

The seat of the Shivagakomarpaj Lineage in Chiang Mai, the Thai Massage School Shivagakomarpaj (fondly known as the "Old Medicine Hospital") is the source of the knowledge of most practitioners, teachers, and schools in the Western world in one form or another. In the year that this second edition of the *Thai Massage Workbook* is being published, the school is celebrating its **50**th anniversary. Founded by the late Ajahn ("Master") Sintorn Chaichakan, the Old Medicine Hospital has grown from humble beginnings to become one of the most prestigious schools in all of Thailand (see details in Chapter **1**).

Classes at the Old Medicine Hospital range from a beginning course through multiple levels of professional training. Classes in Thai herbal massage, Thai foot massage, and other modalities are also provided on a rotating schedule. The Old Medicine Hospital has the distinction of being recognized by all major massage organizations in the United States and Thailand. The school is also accredited to provide continuing education credits for students needing NCBTMB, Yoga Alliance, and other Western professional certifications.

When you travel to the school, allow yourself plenty of time to study. Courses last one to five days; however, the serious student will want to stay for additional classes or internship opportunities. Once you complete a course, you can retake the same course over as often as you would like — either in Thailand or in the US — as a way of deepening your learning and gaining more knowledge.

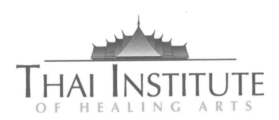

Thai Institute of Healing Arts
www.Thai-Institute.com

To date, the only comprehensive Thai medical education, research, and treatment center outside of Thailand, the Thai Institute of Healing Arts offers a full range of in-depth courses in the Thai medical traditions. The Old Medicine Hospital has designated the Thai Institute as the only official seat of the Shivagakomarpaj Lineage outside of Thailand.

The Thai Institute was founded as a bridge for Westerners to the traditional Thai healing arts. The instructors and staff have all dedicated decades of their life to learning from, or are themselves, native Thai healthcare professionals. The Thai Institute also operates two therapy centers that employ Thais and Westerners offering Thai Massage under the oversight of Traditional Thai Medicine doctors. The organization's therapy, research, and education centers collaborate internally: research is infused into the treatments and the training, while the treatment centers feed clinical data into the research projects and the curriculum. The Thai Institute also provides an interactive online community with access to Thai healing arts practitioners across the world, current research in the field, and resources to start one's own Thai practice — free of charge to the public. Charitable giving is also part of the fabric of the Thai Institute. The institution has initiated multiple projects both in the US and in Thailand that benefit the people of Southeast Asia.

Programs range from a **1**-day Introduction to Thai Massage to a full multi-year Teacher Training Program. A structured progression from the basic levels through to more advanced study includes classes in Traditional Thai Medicine, Thai herbal massage, Thai foot massage, and a certified massage therapy program specializing in Thai Massage that prepares students for the US national certification exam. Continuing education courses are available for students needing NCBTMB, Yoga Alliance, and other professional certification. The Thai Institute is recognized by all major massage organizations in the United States and Thailand (including by the Thai Ministry of Public Health).

44 —) Sa wa deé = Hello or   NOTES   Welcome!
26 —) Polite way → { female → Sawdadee Kaá
5 —) Sounds   Male → Sawadadee Khrab

* Wai → to Respect — to appreciate or to show gratitud.
* Kob Khun → Thank you!
* Kob Khun Mak — Thank you very Much!
* Metta — Kindness — others "be well"
(Thai Institute — 10 year Anniversory.)
(August. 16 – 18, 2013.

Pressure Spectrum

Finger Circle   Thai Chop   a — Stuch
Thumb Circle   Thai Fist   b   Palm
Palm. Circle.   C   Sen work line.
Finger Press   b   Palm
Thumb Press   a. Stuch.
Palm Press
Forearm Roll
Elbow Press
Foot Press
Knee Press
Heel Press.

* Prep & get settle before you put your hands into te client.
* Start Righ side for Male
*   ✓ left side for Female.

Sen = Line (Clearing the stagnation of the body)

OM = Life Force (Where energy flows in the body we field heathy,
energy.

1/20/2013   always ask if there is anything I should know

Four Principles of Thai Massage.

1. – Extremities to Core (out to in)
2. – Feet To head (bottom to Top)
3. – Sen Work, Join Mobilization, Stretches
4. – Balanced Massage.

Day 1 *

Metta
Foot Palm Press ⊚ Knees
9 pts
2 pts.
Bottom Foot Lines "Pluck" toes.
Top Foot Lines ⊚ Notch - Line - ⊚ toes - Traction toes)
Foot Stretch (internal/external)
Ankle Rotation

Repeat on Other Foot

Ankle Stretch ↓↑
Palm Press Legs ⊚ Knees.

Day 2 *

Inside Leg — A B C B A   (2 Lines).
Outside Leg — A B C B A.

Repeat on other Leg

Palm Press Legs ⊚
4 Palm Press

4 Palm Spread (Hip Stretch)
"Paddle Boat"
Finger Press Top Thigh
Thai Fist. Inner thigh
(Lift their Leg w/ My outside Foot)
Leg Traction. one Sure Foot. (Knee 80/20).
Shake the Leg